Counting
Calories

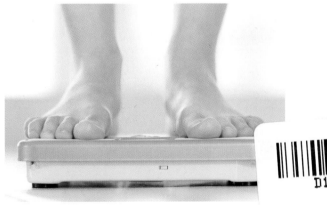

Note: All the nutriti[...]es base[...] on [...]overnment and national health guidelines for healthy eating, and [...] amount an overdose it [...]ommed or [...]ended advice is required, [...]sult your health professional. If you suff[...] [...]e done under the supervision of a health p[...]ofessional. Calorie-counting [...] weight-loss diets are not advisable if you are pregnant unless recommended and super[...] [...]ever follow adult weight-loss or calorie-counting plans.

Publisher & Creative Director: Nick Wells

Copy Editor: Catherine Taylor and Catherine Taylor
and Designer: [...]
Art Direction: [...]
Design: [...]
[...]
Proofreader: [...]

The main references used by the a[...]on, *Dietary Reference Values for Food Energy and Nutrients for the United King[...]on, The Stationary Office, Norwich, 2001; Food Standards Agency, *Manual of Nutrition*, The Stationary Office, Norwich, 2001; McCance, R.A., and Widdowson, E.M., *The Composition of Foods*, Food Standards Agency, The Stationary Office, Norwich, 2002

This is a **FLAME TREE** Book

FLAME TREE PUBLISHING
Crabtree Hall, Crabtree Lane
Fulham, London SW6 6TY
United Kingdom
www.flametreepublishing.com

First published 2011

Copyright © this edition 2014 Flame Tree Publishing Ltd

1 3 5 7 9 10 8 6 4 2
14 16 18 17 15

ISBN: 978-1-78361-329-8

A copy of the CIP data for this book is available from the British Library.

Printed in Singapore

Image credits: © Flame Tree Publishing: 67, 69, 71, 85, 95, 103, 105, 141, 183, 185, 189, 191, 195, 199, 201, 223, 229, 231. **Courtesy Shutterstock.com and © the following photographers**: 1 & 32 & 38, 35t Yuri Arcurs; 3 & 79, 8, 35 b, 43, 93, 99, 137, 155, 163, 164, 205, 219, 235, 237, 239, 241, 243, 249, 251 Monkey Business Images; 4 bonchan; 6 Perrush; 7 -=Vo=-; 9 Karlova Irina; 10 wavebreakmedia ltd; 11 hddigital; 13t, 21, 175 Elena Elisseeva; 13b tonobalaguerf; 15 Andi Berger; 16b AGfoto; 16t Jovan Nikolic; 18 Zaneta Baranowska; 19 Branislav Senic; 20 Dave Nevodka; 22 Jane Rix; 24, 173 Krzysztof Slusarczyk; 26bl, cr Elena Schweitzer; 26tl Valentyn Volkov; 26tr ZoneFatal; 27 Efired; 28 c.; 29 Michael Siegmund; 30t Janina Dierks; 30b pzAxe; 31b emuted; 31t LDprod; 33 Piotr Marcinski; 34t cunaplus; 34b operafotografca; 36, 253 tacar; 47 Zamula Artem; 47, 87 Robyn Mackenzie; 49 Andrea Skjold; 51 Subbotina Anna; 53 KJBevan; 55, 75 Jiri Hera; 57 Juriah Mosin; 61 Borodin Vladimir Vladimirovich; 63 Janet Faye Hastings; 65 MUDU; 73 FikMik; 81 Stephen Mcsweeny; 89, 167 Joe Gough; 97 Kitch Bain; 111 marco mayer; 113 kentoh; 117 Paul Binet; 121 cjorgens; 123 Cathleen A Clapper; 125 dabjola; 129 Ambient Ideas; 131 leungchopan; 133 Yvonne Prancl; 135 Elena Veselova; 143 matka_Wariatka; 145 Studio 1231; 147 Natali Glado; 149 DJM-photo; 153 Lagrima; 157 Patty Orly; 159 Shebeko; 161 Elzbieta Sekowska; 165 Norman Chan; 171 Vania Georgieva; 177 Matthew Benoit; 179 karam Miri; 193 Marina Nabatova; 197 Simone van den Berg; 203 barbaradudzinska; 209 HLPhoto; 213 Christopher Elwell; 215 Studiotouch; 221 Darren Hester; 233 Julian Weber; 245 Irafael; 247 Graça Victoria.

Counting
Calories

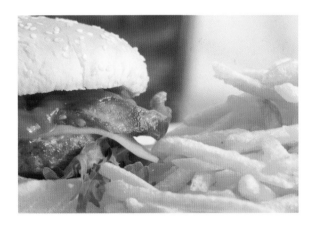

Liz Tucker

**FLAME TREE
PUBLISHING**

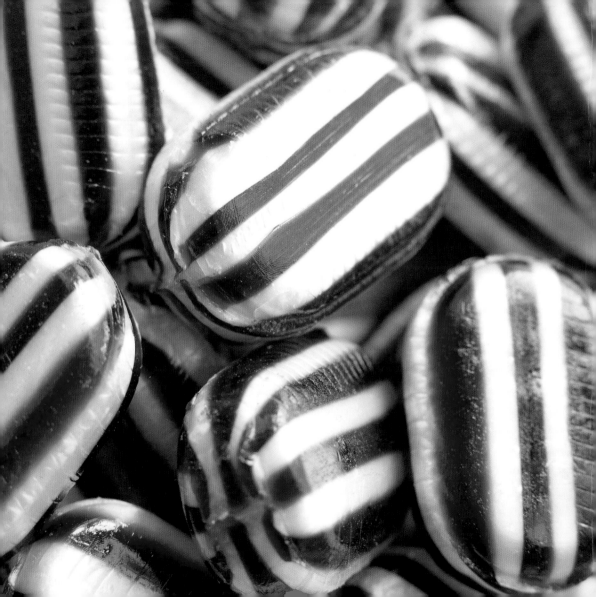

Contents

Introduction

Think of a word most associated with diet and 'calorie' has to be the first to come to most minds. Calorie counting is probably the most recognized form of evaluating food intake, especially when it comes to weight management. Anyone who has ever attempted dieting will have no doubt started by comparing the calorie content of foods they eat, and most diets – no matter how faddy – generally rely on reducing calorie intake to make them effective. Meanwhile, people with high-energy lifestyles, such as sportspeople, are likely to compare calorie content to get the largest number from the most compact source.

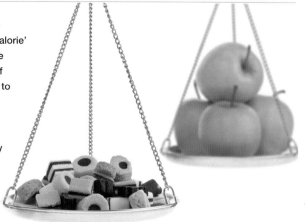

Losing or gaining weight does depend on calorie consumption but this simplistic approach could also lead to a diet that is not necessarily sustainable, satisfying or healthy in the long run.

Being overweight in particular increases your risk of ill health, so it is important to achieve a healthy weight through dieting. But a diet low in calories and fat can also be nutritionally poor, starving you of the energy and essential nutrients needed to stay happy and healthy. An **imbalanced diet** can leave you tired, miserable and constantly craving high-calorie foods – a potential reason why many low-calorie and low-fat diets fail.

Maintaining a sensible weight is an obvious sign of good health, and the key factor in achieving this is a healthy balanced diet. Over the last few decades, nutritional understanding has vastly improved and we now realize that not all calories are the same. Some foods are nutritionally dense, which means they contain a whole range of essential nutrients. Other foods many have the same calorific value but are nutritionally empty, full of fat-forming calories and not a lot else.

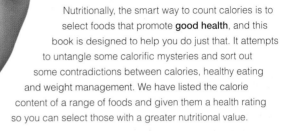

Nutritionally, the smart way to count calories is to select foods that promote **good health**, and this book is designed to help you do just that. It attempts to untangle some calorific mysteries and sort out some contradictions between calories, healthy eating and weight management. We have listed the calorie content of a range of foods and given them a health rating so you can select those with a greater nutritional value.

The food listings are easy to use. Firstly, each food is calculated by **portion size** – a simple way to assess how much you eat. For example, it is easier to imagine a handful of berries than 35 g. Secondly, each food has a calorie and fat content per **100 g/3½ oz** (or ml/fl oz if liquid), so you can compare similar foods. Finally, we have given each food a **health rating**, enabling you to select healthier options. Learn more about how to use this book on pages 36–37.

Note to Reader

It is always advised that professional medical advice is obtained on all personal health matters. The information given here is a guideline only. Any changes to diet or health regime should be done so under the supervision of a health professional. Neither the publisher nor author accepts any legal responsibility for any personal injury or other damage or loss arising from the use or misuse of the information supplied.

What Are Calories?

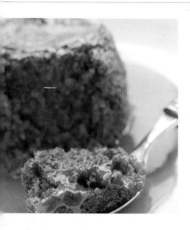

Love Calories

Calories have a bit of a bad reputation. They are those awful little things that either make you put on, or stop you losing, excess weight. Annoyingly, the more indulgent the food, the more calories it seems to have. Let's face it, it's hard to get excited about lettuce, but you can feel the passion oozing out of steamy sticky toffee pudding covered in piping hot custard.

It seems so unfair now, but loving calories has enabled us to survive and become a successful species – we need calories. Think about when humans were first around – food was very hard, even life-threatening, to find. The more calorie-rich the food the better, because by the time you managed to get something to eat, you desperately needed the energy it contained. To give humans the encouragement to search out calorie-rich foods, evolution also added a feeling of **happiness** when food is eaten. Pleasure chemicals in the brain are triggered by food, with more calories generating a bigger energy buzz. Back then, the foods available – such as nuts, seeds and fruit – also had a high nutritional value, so the calorie yearning ultimately provided a diet rich in other essential nutrients.

Over time, we have made it easier to access food and, as pleasure seekers, we have developed foods that have the feelgood rush without any real nutritional quality. Now we hardly need to burn any calories to acquire plenty, and many common calorie sources such as ready meals and snacks do not have the same nutritional backup as our ancestors' foods.

What Do Calories Do?

A **calorie** is just a simple unit of measurement, in this case heat generation – technically, 1 calorie equals the amount of energy required to raise the temperature of 1 gram of water by 1 degree (Celsius).

When our energy demands go up during exercise or under stress, for example, our temperature also rises. To produce the energy needed to cope with this additional exertion, more calories are burnt and this generates the warmth we experience. So a calorie is not a bad thing – it provides **essential energy** without which your body cannot function.

Energy and heat production is measured in many forms, but in food the ones you need to know are either kilocalories (**kcals or 'calories'**) or kilojoules (**kJs**). Most food labels list both but you need to be careful not to mix them up, as kilojoules have a much higher numerical value than kilocalories. Basically, 1 kcal = 4.184 kJs. Kcals are most commonly used to estimate different people's energy requirements and calculate how many calories are needed to maintain a balanced weight, as in the following table.

Daily Estimated Average Energy Requirements

Age	Kcal intake for women	Kcal intake for men
15–18	2110	2755
19–59	1940 (1900 over 50)	2550
60–74	1900	2380 (2330 over 60)

These intakes are overall averages estimated **at rest** or basal metabolic rate (**BMR**). But there are other factors such as climate, state of health and levels of activity that influence how many calories you can consume before weight changes. Exercise is one of the most important, and athletes need much higher calorie intakes to maintain weight and get the additional energy they need to perform at such high endurance levels. Interestingly, the more you weigh, the more calories you burn as every task involves so much more effort. More information on **calorie expenditure** is on pages 29–30 but first it helps to know what energy is used for.

The Role of Energy

We know we need energy to **move** and **think**. However, around two thirds of our daily energy supply is used just running and maintaining internal body parts like the heart, kidneys and digestive system. Most body functions are automatic and we are only aware of them when something goes wrong. It takes great effort to pump blood around constantly, keep the immune system active or digest food, for example. Internal systems are the big energy users and also take priority over your requested energy demands to do things. Low energy levels from poor diet or excess stress, for example, can mean there is not enough to go round. Remember that feeling of fatigue, lack of concentration and co-ordination you get when you are rundown or unhappy. Any health problem or injury pushes up internal energy demands, usually leaving you laid up in bed until it is sorted. It is a simple case of demand outstripping supply. If your aim is to achieve good health and a sustainable weight, getting the **calorific balance** right is much more important than just cutting calories.

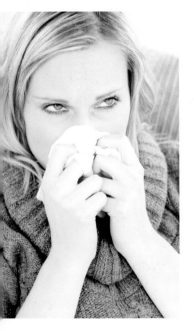

Where Do Calories Come From?

Carbohydrates and fats are the primary energy source. Protein puts body-building and maintenance first, but it can be used for energy, usually when other supplies are temporarily unavailable. Per gram, fat has a much higher calorific value than carbohydrate and protein, making it much easier to gain weight if you eat too much. Alcohol is also high in calories but is often disregarded as a weight-gainer as it is less likely to generate that full feeling. When dieting, it is a common misconception that liquid calories do not count – but they really do!

Calories Per Gram

- 1 gram of carbohydrate or protein = 4 calories
- 1 gram of fat = 9 calories
- 1 gram of alcohol = 7 calories

Our metabolism is used to burn calories into usable energy. **Macro-nutrients** (carbohydrate, protein and fat) are broken down in digestion and transferred to the bloodstream as glucose. Some glucose is combined with oxygen into immediate energy and some is put by for energy later. Any excess ends up being stored in fat cells.

Different carbohydrates are faster or slower at releasing energy. Those closest to glucose, such as sugar, produce an immediate energy rush as they need little processing. More complex carbohydrates, such as wholegrains, involve more digesting, so their energy takes longer to convert and is released in smaller amounts over time. This provides more sustained energy but does not give you such a quick-fix energy buzz!

Fibre

Another type of carbohydrate called non-starch polysaccharide (**NSP**) is more commonly known as 'fibre'. This exists in soluble and insoluble forms derived from fruit, vegetables, grains and pulses. Technically, fibre is not a nutrient but as it has other beneficial roles in the digestive process, it is essential as part of a healthy diet.

Nutritional components other than macro-nutrients are covered later (page 22) but first let's get to know more about fat.

Fat and Calories

There are two obvious types of fat: the fat (fatty acids) in food we eat and the fat we store in internal fat cells. The fat we eat is simply the fat other food sources have stored for their own energy use. Plant products such as vegetables and fruit generally do not contain much fat because they do not have muscle power or brain function. But there is fat in **nuts and seeds** because they need energy to germinate and grow. **Dairy products** also contain fat because their purpose is to rear young.

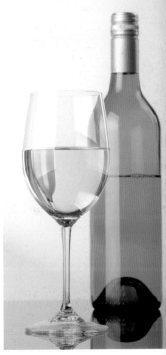

Macro-nutrients Explained

Macro-nutrients	Groups	Role	Rich food sources
Carbohydrates	**Sugars** – e.g. fructose, sucrose, glucose, lactose	Energy supply – fast release	Fruit, sweets, pastries, chocolate, puds
	Starch **See also 'fibre', page 11**	Energy supply – slow release	Vegetables, wholegrains, cereals, pulses
Fats (fatty acids)	**Saturated**	Energy supply; negative effect on health in excess	Meat, dairy, coconut, palm oil
	Unsaturated Including essential fatty acids (EFA) **See also 'trans fats', page 14**	Energy source, but some EFAs, e.g. Omega-3, also vital in body maintenance and function	Nuts, seeds, oily fish, avocado, vegetable oils
Proteins	Around 20 amino acids make a wide range of proteins – individual foods can have proteins unique to them	All protein has primary role in body function, repair and growth; secondary source of energy	Animal sources – meat, fish, dairy, eggs Vegetable sources – nuts, seeds, pulses

Fat cells are simply storage containers that fill up with potential energy. If we didn't have this storage system we would have to eat constantly, which is not very convenient. We stock up on fat so we have energy supplies on demand, and in theory it is very efficient. Fat cells swell and shrink depending on our calorific intake and energy output, changing our size and shape in the process.

Fat Storage

Fast-release carbohydrates may provide quick energy, but cause spikes and troughs in blood sugar levels that ultimately lead to a **craving for more** foods that contain fast-release carbs – this overeating, combined with the fact that these foods are also likely to be fatty and high in calories, leads to weight gain. **Slow-release carbohydrates** are much better, as they provide small amounts of energy over time, so you get a small but steady supply which is more likely to be utilized for energy and less likely to be stored as fat.

Saturated fats are more likely to be stored as fat than essential fatty acids such as **Omega-3**. Like protein, essential fatty acids have a primary body function aside from providing energy, so they are more likely to be put to work rather than stored as fat.

'Good' and 'Bad' Fat

You will put on weight if you consume too much fat whether saturated or unsaturated. While being overweight is unhealthy in itself, it is also important to be aware of the additional health implications of consuming too much saturated fat. Saturated fat is the main dietary cause of high blood cholesterol and has been linked to increased risk of **cardiovascular diseases** and some

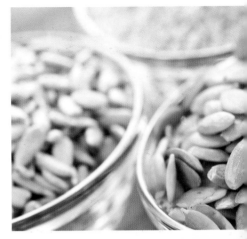

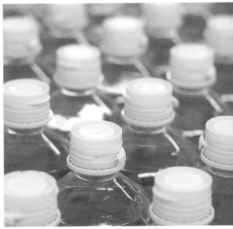

serious long-term health problems. Meanwhile, unsaturated fats can help lower total cholesterol – when eaten as part of a balanced diet.

It should also be noted that, although natural unsaturated fatty acids are generally found in healthier 'cis' form, the process of hydrogenation can transform them into saturated fats, and *partial* hydrogenation produces **'trans fats'**, which, despite being 'unsaturated', are even unhealthier than saturated fats. The key thing to do is avoid any food labelled as containing ingredients that are **hydrogenated** or **partially hydrogenated**, such as processed foods like sweets and biscuits and some margarines, but also beware of unlabelled food such as takeaways and deep-fried food.

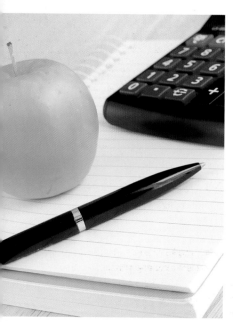

Calorie Count

When it comes to weight, here's the dilemma. Our energy comes from calories, but too many will add weight and too few puts us on a go-slow. Counting calorie intake provides a calculated sum that you can decide to either raise or reduce. If you want to lose weight, fat stores have to be considered. This is how a **calorie-controlled diet** works: put less in and you are forced to use up stored supplies. Cutting down calories from any food will encourage weight loss, but this is not always good nutritionally. Cut down calorific intake too quickly and your body panics, wondering how it will keep everything going with less. Even converting food or stored fat into energy involves lots of energy and nutrition, so to achieve a healthy weight there always needs to be enough resources available.

A diet is unlikely to be sustainable if it is too low in **calories** and also **essential nutrients**. With a low energy intake, cravings for quick-fix sugary and fatty foods are much more likely. Even just thinking about starting a starvation diet puts your brain into sabotage mode and food suddenly becomes obsessive. Your brain thinks 'why go to all that effort converting fat when there is a bag of biscuits in the cupboard?' Even if energy intake is good, without a rich nutritional intake there will not be the resources to process it. Diet deficiencies can generate yo-yo periods of eating too much or too little – and either way, energy levels remain low, leaving you feeling tired and unhappy.

Calories – Different or All the Same?

Biologically, a calorie is a calorie, but nutritionally calories are not all the same. From a health point of view, if you can only consume a certain number it is important that you make every one count. **Good health** and **weight management** go hand in hand. Changing your diet without considering the nutritional impact can leave you feeling tired, miserable, unwell and unlikely to continue. A satisfying diet also has to provide the nutrition your body needs to function effectively, which is why it is so important to consider the calorie source. A calorie may be the same in any food, but nutritionally it can make the difference between a healthy and happy body and one that is constantly exhausted and unwell. Emotionally, not being in control of something seemingly simple like your food intake can destroy confidence and generate a negative relationship with food.

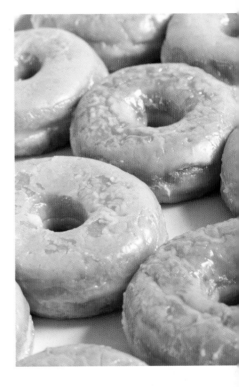

Empty or Dense?

Although calorie counting is an established way of dieting, it has a reputation of being frustratingly difficult to sustain. High-calorie foods are adored but labelled as bad and naughty, making them more appealing. Conversely, low-calorie foods are perceived as dull and boring but with a virtuous halo of goodness, even if nutritionally they are not that good. Selecting nutritionally rich calories from a healthier range of foods can be a much more pleasurable experience than choosing foods by calorie content alone.

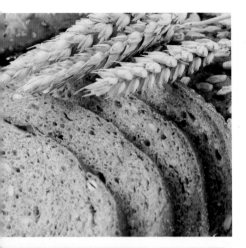

The healthiest calories come from foods with a high **nutritional density**. Nutritional density is measured as nutritional richness per 100 g. This simply means the nutritional content is matched to weight. Foods packed full of nutrients in a compact form are the most nutritionally dense. For example, seeds have a high nutritional density as loads of nutrients are crammed into a small package. This also means they have a high calorific value, but just a small amount has a lot of nutrition. A doughnut, for example, might have a similar calorie value but, nutritionally, it is a dessert. You could eat loads and still not match the nutritional density of a few seeds. This is referred to as empty calories – a high calorific value but nutritionally very poor. Therefore it is healthier to fill your calorie quota with nutritionally dense foods than waste precious calories on empty foods.

Calorie Counter or Healthy Eater?

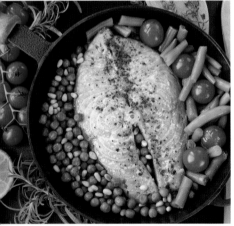

It is probably no surprise to learn that the most nutritionally dense foods are **pure, natural foods** such as vegetables, fish, nuts, seeds, wholegrains and eggs. It's even less of a shock to discover foods most likely to contain empty calories are processed and refined foods such as fast food, ready meals, snacks, alcohol and fizzy drinks. Many empty-calorie foods are also more likely to contain less-healthy nutritional components such as saturated or trans fats, additives and excess salt. Not only are nutritionally dense foods healthier but, when combined, they can also make delicious and **satisfying meals**. Home-made pizza, oven-cooked chips and burgers are easy to make from healthy ingredients at a comparative cost, and taste so much better.

Examples of Nutritionally Dense and Empty Calories

	Typical empty-calorie food	Nutritionally dense food
Snacks	Sweets, biscuits, cakes, crisps	Nuts, seeds, fruit
Meals	Takeaways, ready meals, fast food	Roast dinner, casseroles, stir-fry, risotto
Drinks	Fizzy drinks, alcohol, frothy coffee	Sugar-free fruit juice and squash, smoothies
Breakfasts	Pastries, fried sausages in white bap, fry-up with white bread	Wholegrain bread or cereal, fruit, natural yogurt, grill-up with wholemeal bread

Choosing nutritionally dense foods rather than empty-calorie ones does not mean you need to give up food you love. For example, if you are a chocoholic, select dark chocolate and mix with dried fruit, nuts and seeds. Instead of a fast-food milkshake, make one at home with real fruit. The chances are you will prefer the taste and, because it is **richer**, be satisfied with less.

Which One Are You?

Healthy Eater	Calorie Counter
Selects food for its nutritional value	Selects food for its calorie content
Knows the basic nutrition in food	Knows the calorie content of most food
Knows how to create balanced meals	Sets calorie targets for each meal
Makes meals to share with everyone	Eats separate meals and longs to eat like everyone else
Enjoys treats and indulgences	Feels guilty about having treats and indulgences but can't resist them anyway
Eats regularly or when they are hungry	Thinks about food all the time

Although calorie intake is an important factor in weight management, it is more effective when combined with a nutritionally rich diet. Basically, become both a healthy eater and a calorie counter. Sounds complicated? It could not be more simple. Once you have a basic understanding of a healthy diet, eating for health and weight management becomes **instinctive** rather than difficult.

A Healthy Diet

Food – More Than Fuel

Food is essential. At a basic level, we all know food is our fuel source but some of us do not realize we are actually made and run from the nutritional components we get from eating. Every bit of your body – from manufacture to maintenance – is totally reliant on **nutrients**. Every cellular structure, including bones, muscles, organs, blood and brain, is made from and run on nutrients only found in our diet. Bodily functions will not occur without a mix of vitamins and minerals. It seems obvious but we need a healthy, varied, balanced diet to make a healthy body. There is no way round it – if you don't put in the right mix of nutrients, it will be much harder for your body to function, which also makes it difficult for you to stay happy and healthy.

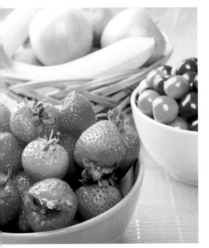

Nutrients generally have multiple roles that involve interaction with a range of other nutrients. Individual nutrients in isolation rarely work effectively, which is why **balance** is so important. Repeatedly eating the same food will give you an overload in some nutrients and a deficiency in others, reducing nutrient efficiency and adding internal problems of toxicity, storage and disposal. This is where nutritionally dense calories win over empty ones. If you want plenty of sustained energy you also need the nutritional components that manufacture it.

Easier Said Than Done

This is the deal. Your body will keep all your internal systems up and running, cope with constant change, keep you safe, offer the best advice, put up with your environment and deal with your constant demands. Your role is simply to give it the right resources and circumstances to enable it to do just that. It sounds simple but life can often conspire against our attempts to follow a healthier route. For example, if you have a problem at home or work, you worry more, comfort-eat and put weight on. Then you feel tired but hungry all the time, so you eat more. This means you feel unhappy about how you look and so you stop going out. Eating comfort food becomes your main source of pleasure, and it becomes extremely difficult to stop.

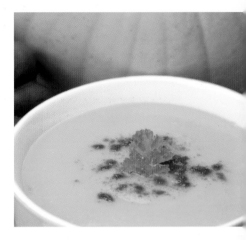

This example shows how one external reaction can destabilize your weight, undermine your internal health and emotionally make you less able to resolve that initial problem. It also demonstrates the individuality of a problem: someone else under stress could forget to eat, lose weight and become malnourished. What remains the same is the potential consequence of poor health at a time when you really need additional resources to cope.

Variety is the Spice of Life

What you put into your body has a huge effect on its ability to function, manage and maintain. We all know we need **food** and **water** to survive, but it cannot be just any old food or fluid if you also want to stay fit and healthy. Your body has thousands of different components that need constant maintenance and a vast array of tasks to carry out, and this requires a quantity of energy and nutrients selected from a varied and balanced diet. Forget some magical **superfood** – no one food item contains all the nutrients we need.

Why We Need Variety and Balance
- Eating lots of one type of food and neglecting others is nutritionally pointless. Nutrients rarely work independently and eating the same foods over and over again will also deprive your body of other essential nutrients.
- Eating a varied diet reduces the likelihood of **food sensitivities**.
- Eating **seasonally** provides a more natural diet, and one your body is more accustomed to.
- **Variety** makes our diet more satisfying, so we are less likely to overeat.

Assess Your Diet's Variety

We often think we eat a whole variety of food, but at a basic level it can be very repetitive. It is more likely to be the same basic foods processed in a different way. This makes our tastebuds less responsive and we end up eating without really tasting and becoming less aware of when to stop.

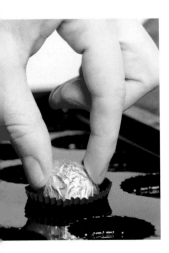

For example, western diets are generally high in **wheat** and **dairy**. Wheat and dairy have been a perfectly healthy staple food for generations, but more recently they have been found in more refined and processed foods, which are also more likely to be high in fat, sugar and salt but low in nutrition. If you look around a supermarket at the vast array of food available, it is easy to be overwhelmed with the choice but if you look at the basic ingredients, much of it is actually not that different. If you related this to a typical diet, it would be something like this:

- Bowl of cereal and tea for breakfast
- Mid-morning latte and biscuit snack
- Sandwich and yogurt for lunch
- Afternoon chocolate fix
- Pasta in a creamy sauce with garlic bread, followed by ice cream and a glass or two of wine for supper
- Savoury snacks to nibble in front of the TV with another glass of wine

This may look like lots of different foods but at basic ingredient level it can be summed up as mainly wheat and dairy washed down with caffeine and alcohol. It must be stressed that neither wheat nor dairy are 'bad' foods. In wholegrain form, wheat is a complex carbohydrate, rich in B vitamins and full of fibre. Similarly, milk is one of the best sources of calcium, especially for pre-menopausal women. However, in this diet they are not only in excess but also in less nutritionally rich forms. Anyone cutting wheat and dairy out of this diet will be forced to eat not only a more **varied** diet but also a more nutritionally **balanced** one as vegetables, seeds, alternative wholegrains and fruit are some of the few things left to eat. This change of diet could result in weight loss and more energy, but this is not because of an 'allergy' to wheat and dairy. The change is much more likely due to a healthier nutritional re-balancing.

Forget 'Good' or 'Bad'

For healthy eating, forget about classifying foods as **good** or **bad** and think more about too much or too little for too long. If you class something as good then, theoretically, the more you eat, the healthier it will be. Bad, on the other hand, is sinful and needs to be avoided at all costs. In reality, all foods have some good components and others that are either of no value or potentially damaging in large quantities. For example, you may lose a lot of weight quickly on a diet of nothing but fruit and salad but it is unlikely to be sustainable, healthy or enjoyable in the long term.

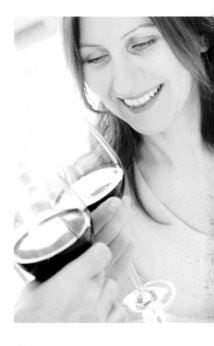

Psychologically, the good/bad food mindset makes it much harder to eat healthily or maintain a balanced weight. Yes, some foods are better to eat than others because they have a much higher nutritional density, but a **balanced diet** accounts for all your requirements in the right quantities. That means you can continue to enjoy your favourite foods, so you shouldn't feel deprived. In a balanced diet, so-called bad foods such as chocolate and red wine are perfectly good. On the other hand, a diet of nothing but chocolate and red wine is not at all good. In fact, if you were forced to follow this regime, it would not be long before vegetable cravings kicked in!

What Nutrients Do

To summarize, there are two main reasons why we need food. Firstly, it gives us **energy**, and secondly it helps to **build** and **maintain** body parts and make everything function internally. Most foods contain a combination of both energy and body-building nutrients but in different variations, quantities and ratios. Sugar is the most basic and simple food as its only nutritional value is as an energy source. But before you all start thinking 'and therefore it must be bad', find yourself stuck up a mountain and sugar could be a lifesaver. As sugar is found in some amount in most foods, adding it to our diet is not really necessary, but that doesn't mean we can't enjoy a little bit if we fancy.

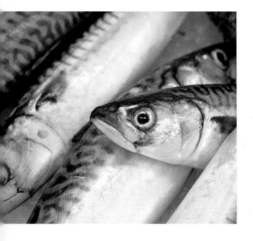

Micro-nutrients

We have already looked at the role of macro-nutrients (pages 11–12) but there are other nutrients we need in much smaller quantities. These are called **micro-nutrients**. Although micro-nutrients are often only required in trace amounts, they have a massive role to perform. **Minerals** and **vitamins** are the key micro-nutrients and collectively they are responsible for a wide range of jobs from energy production to digestion to making teeth and bones. There are also other nutritional components in food that play a health role – these are referred to as active food chemicals (**AFCs**). AFCs, such as flavonols, phytosterols, carotenoids and prebiotics, are nutritional assistants that provide a long list of functions including maintaining digestive health, boosting immunity and regulating cholesterol.

Nutritionally Confused?

With all these macro and micro-nutrients, AFCs and NSPs, managing a healthy balanced diet is beginning to sound a bit too complicated. Thankfully, **nature** keeps it simple by putting a whole combination of these nutrients in the same nutritionally dense foods. When healthy eating is mentioned, you will keep coming back to the same foods that are high in a whole variety of nutrients, such as nuts, seeds, wholegrains, fruit, meat, fish, eggs and dairy – in fact all basic, natural ingredients that have always been the basis of a healthy diet. For example, seeds contain a wide range of nutrients, including all the macros, a good mix of micros, fibre and a variety of AFCs.

And you don't need to cross the world to find rare so-called antioxidant-rich **superfoods** when blackcurrants and berries are so rich in nutrients and can be grown almost anywhere. As there is no one food that contains everything you need in the ratio you need, the key to a healthy diet is to mix and match your natural food groups. There are more details on balancing your diet in the next section, but first let's get to know the natural food groups a bit better.

Natural Food Groups

Vegetables

Vegetables are great: they are packed full of a whole range of nutrients and are generally low in fat and calories. For healthy eating, it is best to divide veg into two groups:

- **Coloured veg** This includes, not surprisingly, anything red, green, orange, purple, yellow – the more vivid, the better! Green leafy veg, squashes, beetroot, carrots, peppers; the list is long and lovely. These should account for a big part of your diet as they are packed full of nutrition. When we think about **'5 a day'**, at least three of these should be coloured veg.

- **Starch veg** A smaller group that includes potatoes and pulses such as lentils and kidney beans. They are also nutritionally good but have a higher carbohydrate and calorie value, so they are great if you need energy, but should be eaten in moderation if you want to lose weight.

Meat

Lean meat, such as skinless turkey and chicken and non-fatty red meat, is an excellent source of protein, vitamins and minerals. The meats you need to watch are fatty cuts, and especially processed meats such as burgers, sausages and pâtés, as generally they have more saturated fat and fewer micro-nutrients, making their calories more likely to be empty.

Fish and Seafood

Seafood and fish are great sources of nutrients. Fish can be divided into two groups:

- **Oily fish** A great source of essential fatty acids, especially **Omega-3** oils, oily fish include salmon, trout and mackerel. Although higher in calories than white fish, they are generally more nutritionally dense. Tuna is also an oily fish, but be aware that, when canned, it loses its Omega-3 content.

- **White fish** A great source of low-fat protein, examples of white fish are cod and haddock. As with meat, the things it gets processed with can make it less healthy.

Eggs

Eggs contain a wide range of nutrients. Basically, an egg is just a big cell designed purely for growth and development, so it contains all the nutrients needed to carry out that very complex process.

Dairy

Milk is designed for growth and development, so it is nutritionally rich, but its products can have a high fat content. Skimmed milk actually has more calcium than full fat, but less **Vitamin D** – so once again it is about balance.

Fruit

Fruit and vegetables are often grouped under the same nutritional status but veg generally has a wider range of nutrients and much less sugar. The fruit is the bit the plant wants us to eat, so it is deliberately sweet. Nutrients are crammed in the seed or nut to aid growth. However, fruit still has plenty of nutritional value and provides a great source of energy. It is also a healthier option for those with a **sweet tooth**.

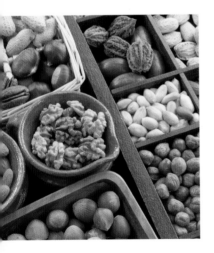

Nuts and Seeds

Dieters often avoid nuts and seeds because they are high in calories and fat, but they also have some of the highest nutritional densities. They are the plant version of an egg as they are responsible for the germination of a new plant, so they are packed full of nutrients including fibre, essential fatty acids and protein. Their calories are much more satisfying than more empty-calorie snacks, filling you up sooner so that you will snack less often.

Cereals

There are a wide range of grains that provide a main source of carbohydrate in the diet, including oats, rye and rice. Wholegrains contain minerals, vitamins and fibre, but these are often removed in refining to produce white flours and breads. Mass-produced confectionery, pastries and ready meals using refined grains are more likely to contain empty calories.

Water

Although not a nutrient, **water** is essential for good health, so it is worth mentioning. A large proportion of our body is water, and it is constantly being used, so it needs replacing. A lot of our fluid intake today is in the form of tea, coffee, fizzy drinks and alcohol, which can also have a high empty-calorie content.

Processed Foods

Natural foods are all so simple and basic they don't need an ingredient label. Anything mixed together to make a final product has to be processed in some way and neither the processing or the end product is necessarily unhealthy. Some processed foods are made from natural, nutritionally valuable basic ingredients – and the list is growing. There is no reason why we have to sacrifice convenience for healthy foods. Healthier snacks, wholegrain breads and the like are now much more readily available, but unfortunately the majority of processed foods are **high in calories** and have little other nutritional value. Refining grain on the whole reduces its health rating and affects the impact it has on blood glucose. For example, some white flour can be so refined it can produce a similar high peak effect on blood glucose levels to sugar.

What's on the List?

The easiest way to select healthier options is to look at the **label**. Generally, the shorter the list, the better, especially if it is a list of ingredients that you recognize rather than a long list of numbers and weird names.

Healthy Diet Ratio

From an energy point of view, the standard dietary advice for a balanced diet is 50% carbohydrates, 35% fat and 15% protein.

Macro-nutrient Percentage Ratio of Daily Energy Intake

Carbohydrate	50% (maximum 10% as added sugar)
Fat	35% (minimum 18% unsaturated fat, maximum 2% trans fats)
Protein	15%

Initially this seems simple but in reality all foods have a combination of fats, proteins and/or carbohydrates in them and I doubt if even the most qualified nutritionist would be able to reel off each one, or would even bother to. For example, nuts are often classed as a protein and oats as a carbohydrate, but they both contain all the macro-nutrients: **carbohydrate**, **fat** and **protein**. Apart from a few, such as sugar, most foods do not fit into one category alone.

One of the rules of healthy eating is not to get obsessive about food, desperately trying to match nutrient with food item. It is much easier to work directly with the natural food groups.

Handed On A Plate

Professional health guidelines demonstrate dietary balance with an **'eatwell'** plate or food pyramid. Here's how it works. Firstly, divide the natural foods into three: groups A, B and C.

- **A** is coloured vegetables – that is, all veg apart from potatoes and pulses. This is what I refer to as the 'free range' category and should make up the major part of your diet.
- **B** is starchy vegetables, pulses, fruit and cereals that are predominately carbohydrate.
- **C** is meat, fish, eggs, dairy, nuts and seeds, which are rich sources of protein.

Then think of a plate and divide it into sections, the proportionate sizes of which depend on your aims:

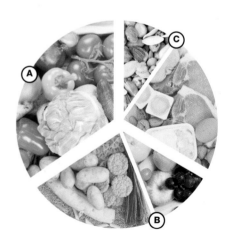

- **For a healthy maintenance diet**, there should be an equal-sized section each for the A, B and C foods (pictured), and the various foods within those sections should be balanced – in other words, section C cannot be made up entirely of dairy foods!
- **For weight loss**, section A could be increased to half the plate, leaving a quarter each for B and C.
- **If you need to gain weight**, you need a bigger plate!

This is a very simple way of getting an idea of **nutritional balance**. Obviously, milk or yogurt is a bit messy on a plate, but you can still visualize the quantity needed. If you are preparing a meal, you can divide the food before you prepare it. Do this exercise on an average meal and it can be quite a surprise how different the ratio is to your usual portions, especially when it comes to coloured veg.

Moving your diet towards natural, basic foods is a great move for your health and weight management, even if you do not get the ratio spot on. Not only will you be eating more nutritionally valuable food, it is also more likely to be **ecologically** and **ethically** sound. It may even encourage you to grow your own, and there is nothing more delicious and ecologically favourable than that.

The 90% Rule

Food should be a **pleasure**, and there is no getting away from the fact that, although we are reaping the benefits of loads of energy and a balanced weight from following a natural healthy diet, we still love some foods that have empty calories. Being happy with your food is all part and parcel of eating healthily, and a good way to maintain the balance is to follow the 90% rule. If **90%** of your diet is from the natural food groups, then you could enjoy the odd takeaway, cream cake or double choc chip dessert. Over time you may find that they become less appealing anyway, so there is no harm in doing the odd experiment every now and then!

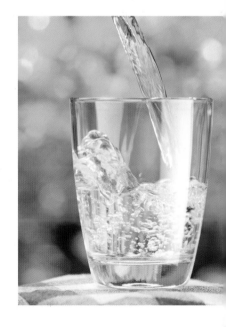

What About Water?

The 90% ratio is also very good for working out if you are drinking enough **water**. It is all very well drinking a litre a day, but that can be ruined if you also have 10 cups of coffee and a bottle of wine. If you follow the 90% rule and make 90% of your fluid intake water, then you can enjoy a glass of wine or a cup of coffee without going too far off balance.

Controlling Your Weight

Weight and Health

When it comes to diet, think firstly about health, and weight will fall into place. The potential risks over time of developing serious health conditions such as heart disease and diabetes rise dramatically with increasing weight. Even in a relatively short time there can be a noticeable impact on **energy levels** and overall state of health. As weight goes on, it is easy to lose confidence, making you less inspired to do new and interesting things. If this picture of weight gain is so gloomy, why do we find it so difficult to motivate ourselves in a healthier direction?

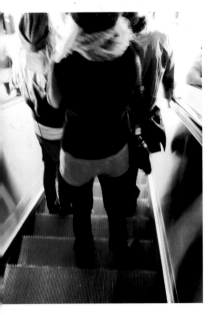

Weight Influences

Theoretically, the more calories we put in, the more energy we produce. But it seems in reality that the more you eat, the more exhausted you feel, generating compulsive cravings for foods we know will add more weight. To lose weight we simply have to eat less and exercise more, but in reality, matching calorie intake to energy output is not that simple. Balancing **intake** and **output** is the key to managing weight effectively but in order to achieve this we need to find out what other factors are getting in the way.

Keep Moving

What we eat dictates how good our energy levels are, and a diet rich in nutritious food is more likely to make you want to get up and go. Unfortunately, lifestyles today do not make it that easy. Humans have until relatively recently had to rely on their own steam to get things done. Over time we have developed labour-saving devices, so although days managing family and work are long, energy outputs have fallen. It seems we are too busy not being active to have the time to be active.

Unfortunately, the brain will always suggest the easiest option unless you can convince it otherwise. For example, if you need an energy boost it prefers to remind you of that packet of biscuits in the cupboard than go to the trouble of converting fat. Similarly, given the option of car or foot, the keys are in your hand before you know it.

Find the Incentive

If you can prove you are more likely to get **enjoyment** or **satisfaction** from a new healthier approach then you will get inner encouragement to carry on. As with unsustainable dull and boring diets, activity has to have purpose and a positive end result, and one of the best is feeling fit and healthy. If you have a busy life, being fit makes it more manageable, so getting more active can make life easier in the long run.

You do not need to set aside a specific time to do exercise – your **daily routine** can be very active. The simplest way to assess your activity level is to carry a step-meter and aim for 10,000 steps a day.

Good things about being active:

- You get the same sort of **feelgood** buzz you get from high-calorie foods, so experience fewer cravings.
- It helps you manage **stress** and gives you time out to relax.
- It makes you **happier** and more in control.
- You can eat more and still maintain a balanced **weight**.

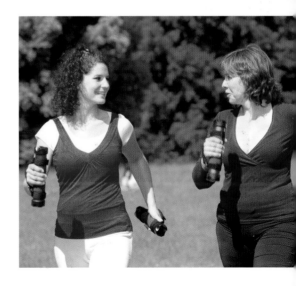

Activity Calorie Burner

On page 9 there is a basic table of energy requirements at rest. If you add **activity**, then energy requirements go up – as shown in the table overleaf. Therefore, if you keep your calorie intake the same and exercise more, you will lose weight. If you find it hard to maintain your weight, increasing activity will give you extra calories to make your diet more sustainable.

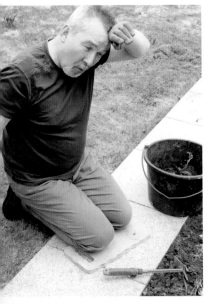

Activity	Kcals burnt in 30 minutes
Walking moderately	105
Walking on stairs	195
Gardening	125
Dancing	135
Jogging	195

As you can see, daily activities burn plenty of calories so you can scrap that gym membership if you have no time to use it and incorporate activity into things you have to or want to do. Forget exercise as a time-consuming extra to living and think more about being active in life.

On A Diet – Honestly?

If you want to improve your diet, the first step is to find out how much you are currently eating. Doing a simple five-day **food diary** logging everything you eat and drink will enable you to assess and isolate some of the key problem areas. Some people tell me they eat healthily but are still tired and overweight. The biggest problem I find with food diaries is that they are often not that accurate, as it can be really hard to admit you eat unhealthily. To be successful you must be **honest** about including everything – it can be a great way to shock you into action!

Why Your Diet May Not Be As Healthy As You Think

Irregular Eating

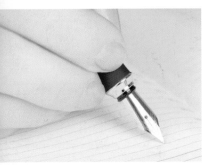

Having no set eating pattern encourages your body to hoard energy supplies and filter out only the bare minimum, as it doesn't know when the next lot is coming. When food does appear, your instinct will be to eat as much as possible.

Double Eating

You have packed a low-calorie salad for lunch, but by lunchtime you have a crisp craving. You resist and eat the salad but still have cravings, so you have a bagful mid-afternoon. Asked what you had for lunch, you say 'Oh, just a salad'. Finishing off leftovers, eating out and nicking off someone else's plate are common examples of double eating. Unplanned calories may not be written on your diet plan but they still count.

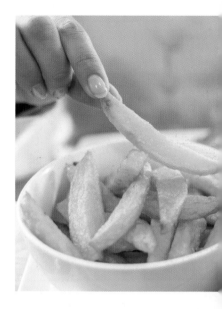

Portion Sizes

Portion sizes have grown dramatically over the last few decades and bear little resemblance to the **recommended guidelines**, which look something like this:

- Serving of **vegetables** = size of a fist
- Serving of **cheese** = one domino piece
- Serving of **meat** or **fish** = deck of cards
- Serving of **peanut butter** = tip of your thumb
- Average **baked potato** = computer mouse
- Serving of **cereal** = compact disc
- Serving of **rice** or **pasta** = a rounded handful

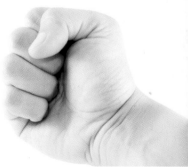

Glasses, plates and packet sizes have all got bigger, making it harder to estimate or allocate the right amount. This is why we list portion sizes in the food tables. Initially it is worth measuring your portion size against those listed here. Visually it is easy to imagine a bowl or handful, but you need to check your cubic capacity matches ours (see listing on page 37).

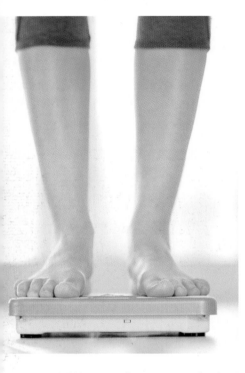

Stress

From the busy body's point of view, foods high in calories, sugar and fat give immediate energy with little processing so you are more likely to crave them under stress. Eating for stress is not just about energy; with any ongoing anxiety or negative event, food can become a compulsive rare source of pleasure and satisfaction.

Are You The Right Weight?

Even if we have a perfectly healthy weight and attractive body we can still believe we are overweight. Being stick-thin is not necessarily healthy, so the key is to find a **healthy weight** you are comfortable with. There are various ways of estimating if your weight is healthy. The simplest ones are waist-to-height, waist-to-hip and height-to-weight (BMI) comparisons. Remember that 1 inch = 2.5 cm, 12 inches (1 ft) = 0.3 m, 1 lb (16 oz) = 0.45 kg, and 1 stone/14 lb = 6.35 kg.

Waist-to-height ratio calculation

- Divide your **waist** measurement by your **height** in centimetres.
- For example, 69 cm waist ÷ 172 cm height = 0.4.
- A figure of 0.4 to 0.5 (40–50 %) is generally considered healthy.

Waist-to-hip ratio calculation

- Divide **waist** measurement by **hip** measurement in centimetres.
- For example, 69 cm waist ÷ 92 cm hip = 0.75.
- For men, the ratio should be under 0.90. For women, it should be under 0.85.

People with a classic 'apple' shape are more likely to have higher totals, and this is matched to an increased risk of heart disease.

Height-to-weight, also known as Body Mass Index (BMI)

First, square your **height** in metres, then divide your **weight** in kilograms by the squared **height** sum. For example, for someone 1.75 metres tall and weighing 65 kilograms: 1.75 m x 1.75 m = 3.06; 65 ÷ 3.06 = BMI of 21.24. Using the chart below, you can estimate your weight status:

Below 18.5	Underweight
18.5–24.9	Normal
25–29.9	Overweight
30 and above	Obese

Too Sporty?

Unfortunately, **BMI** is not accurate in some circumstances. Sportspeople often have overweight or even obese BMIs because of their muscle mass, which pushes up their weight. If you are this fit, it can be hard to get the calories you need. Some endurance athletes need two or even three times the average daily calorific intake and many high-calorie foods are full of empty calories. These may well boost energy in the short term, but nutritionally dense calories provide a more **consistent** supply of energy over time while keeping your body healthy.

A Healthier Way to Cut Calories

The healthiest way to lose weight is slowly and steadily. Starvation puts your body into an energy-loss panic and increases the risk of nutritional deficiencies.

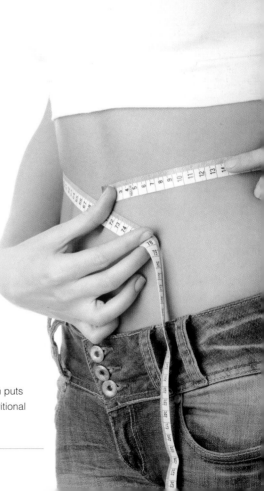

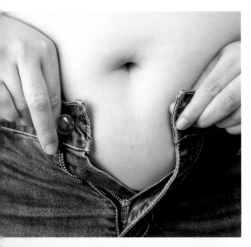

If You Need to Lose More than 4 Kg

If this is the case, your calorie intake could be well above average and cutting to the recommended amount straight away may be too drastic. Your food diary will help you to pinpoint the easiest calories to cut or replace with more nutritionally dense foods. This enables you to set a more **achievable** calorie target.

Cutting 500 calories a day loses about 1 pound (0.45 kg) a week. This may not seem much but this rate is likely to be burning stored fat. If you lose weight too quickly, fluid and muscle tissue could be lost as well.

If You Want to Lose Less than 4 Kg

In this case, your existing calorie intake may match or be up to 500 calories over the recommended amount. If this is the case then the key considerations are converting to nutritionally dense foods and increasing activity levels rather than reducing calories.

Eating For Ever Action Plan

When making healthier changes in your life, success is all in the **planning**. Points you need to consider before you start:

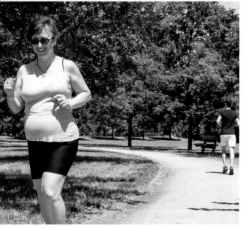

- Set a **realistic** timescale with small, regular, achievable goals.
- Address current **limitations** such as a busy job or young children.

- Include healthy **rewards** like a day out or a new outfit.
- Be **honest** and avoid denial.
- Build in satisfying **activities** that you look forward to doing.
- Be **flexible** – you may need to experiment to find what suits you.

Steps To Success

Assess your existing diet How balanced and varied is it? What proportion of natural foods do you really eat? What's your nutritional ratio?

Assess your understanding of a healthy diet
How aware are you of what you eat? Can you estimate quantities? Can you tell a nutritionally dense food from an empty calorie?

Assess your progress What is and isn't working? How much have you achieved? How can you improve on that?

Assess your attitude Are you being realistic? Can you work with your lifestyle limitations? Can you cope with inevitable setbacks?

Eat For Life

If you make health a priority, it is much easier to get and keep a weight and shape you want for good. We need to eat healthily but this doesn't mean it has to be an ordeal. You can eat lots of highly **nutritious** and **tasty** food and have a happy body that looks great, and there's nothing dull or boring about that!

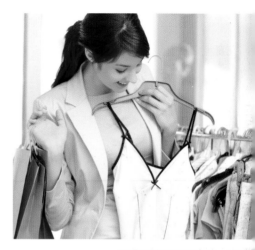

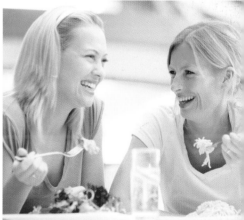

How To Use This Book

The foods in the tables are listed in their natural food groups or groupings similar to shops. When a food fits more than one group, it is listed in one and referenced in any others. There is an alphabetical index as well.

Portion Sizes

The portion sizes used in the book are based on an average standard size bought or served. These may differ from the recommended healthy eating portion guidelines below.

Food	Recommended portion	Food	Recommended portion
Fruit and vegetables	80 g/3 oz	Milk	200 ml/7 fl oz
Meat and fish	100 g/3½ oz	Yoghrt	125 ml/4 fl oz
Cereal or pasta	50 g/2 oz (dry uncooked)	Cheese	30 g/1 oz
Nuts and seeds	28 g/1 oz	Spreads	5 ml/1 tsp
Chocolate	28–30 g/1 oz		

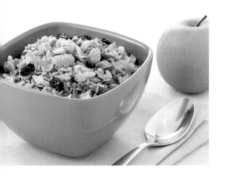

Portion sizes in both weight and serving method are listed where applicable. This makes it easier to **visualize** portions, but you do initially need to **weigh** a sample for comparison, as portions may be very different to your usual serving. Remember that food weights vary (1 tablespoon may hold 40 g of potato, for example, but only 25 g of cabbage).

As bowls, spoons and handfuls have different capacities, standard sizes have been used. To compare your vessels and utensils with the standard sizes, you need a measuring jug and some water. Fill your spoon, glass or bowl with water, then pour it into the jug. Compare your measurements with this table:

Serving method and abbreviation	Standard capacity
Teaspoon (tsp)	5 ml/$\frac{1}{6}$ fl oz
Dessertspoon (dssp)	10 ml/$\frac{1}{3}$ fl oz
Tablespoon (tbsp)	15 ml/$\frac{1}{2}$ fl oz
Cup	220 ml/7$\frac{3}{4}$ fl oz ($\frac{14}{15}$ US cup)
Mug	227 ml/8 fl oz ($\frac{17}{18}$ US cup)
Bowl	300 ml/$\frac{1}{2}$ pint (1$\frac{1}{4}$ US cups)
Tumbler glass	150 ml/$\frac{1}{4}$ pint ($\frac{2}{3}$ US cup)
Wine glass	120 ml/4 fl oz ($\frac{1}{2}$ US cup)
Tall glass	250 ml/8$\frac{3}{4}$ fl oz (1$\frac{2}{5}$ US cup)
Spirit measure	35 ml/1$\frac{1}{4}$ fl oz spirits or 25 ml/1 fl oz liqueurs

Comparisons

Some foods do not have typical serving sizes, so both calories and fat **per 100 g/ml** (3$\frac{1}{2}$ oz/fl oz) are listed. This makes it easier when comparing recipes, menus and foods. Most prepared foods are **based on shop-bought ('retail') or takeaway**. But by combining basic ingredients, you can see how much **healthier home-made** could be.

Figures, Products and Brands

Figures tend to be an **average taken across products**, whereas some are taken from specific brands. Remember to take them as a **guide**, rather than relying on them down to the last calorie. If a brand name is mentioned, this is an **example** of the type of product – the figures given do not necessarily represent the specific nutritional information for that brand.

Health Rating

Each food has an at-a-glance health rating between **1** and **10** (highest is healthiest). This is a subjective assessment based on **nutritional density**, so you can select **healthier options** and be more aware of emptier calories. Remember that one food may have fewer calories, but another may have a higher health rating – do not neglect your health for the sake of cutting a few calories.

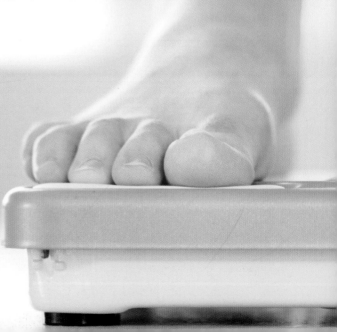

Calorie

Counter

Eggs, Dairy & Fats

	Typical portion	Typical portion size	Calories per portion	Calories per 100 g/ml	Fat per 100 g/ml	Health rating (1–10)
Milk						
Skimmed milk	1 glass	200 ml/7 fl oz	64	**32**	0.2	7
Skimmed milk, pasteurized	1 glass	200 ml/7 fl oz	68	**34**	0.3	7
Skimmed milk, pasteurized, fortified	1 glass	200 ml/7 fl oz	78	**39**	0.1	7
Skimmed milk, UHT	1 glass	200 ml/7 fl oz	54	**27**	0.1	6
Semi-skimmed milk	1 glass	200 ml/7 fl oz	92	**46**	1.7	7
Semi-skimmed milk, pasteurized	1 glass	200 ml/7 fl oz	92	**46**	1.7	7
Semi-skimmed milk, pasteurized, fortified	1 glass	200 ml/7 fl oz	102	**51**	1.6	7
Semi-skimmed milk, UHT	1 glass	200 ml/7 fl oz	92	**46**	1.6	5
Whole milk	1 glass	200 ml/7 fl oz	132	**66**	3.9	6
Whole milk, pasteurized	1 glass	200 ml/7 fl oz	132	**66**	3.9	6
Whole milk, UHT	1 glass	200 ml/7 fl oz	132	**66**	3.9	4
Channel Island milk, whole, pasteurized	1 glass	200 ml/7 fl oz	156	**78**	5.1	5
Channel Island breakfast milk, pasteurized	1 glass	200 ml/7 fl oz	144	**72**	4.7	5
Condensed milk, skimmed, sweetened	1 tbsp	14 g/½ oz	37	**267**	0.2	3
Condensed milk, whole, sweetened	1 tbsp	14 g/½ oz	47	**333**	10.1	2
Dried skimmed milk	2 tbsp	28 g/1 oz	97	**348**	0.6	5
Dried skimmed milk with vegetable fat	2 tbsp	28 g/1 oz	136	**487**	25.9	4
Evaporated milk, whole	1 tbsp	14 g/½ oz	21	**151**	9.4	3

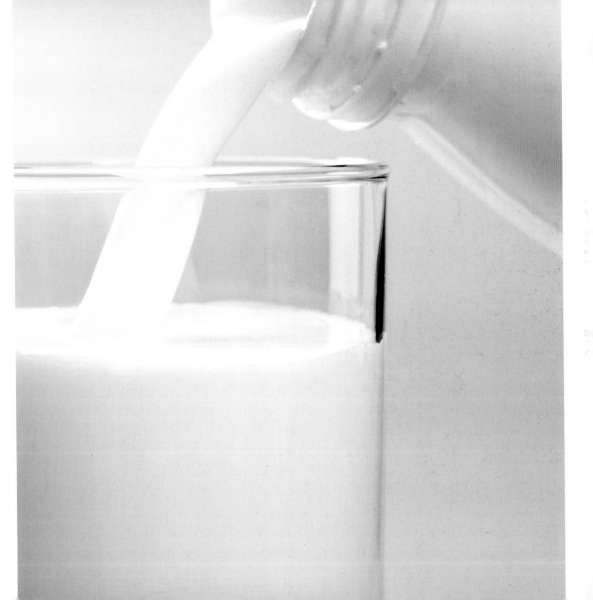

Counting Calories: Eggs, Dairy & Fats

	Typical portion	Typical portion size	Calories per portion	Calories per 100 g/ml	Fat per 100 g/ml	Health rating (1–10)
Evaporated milk, light, 4% fat	1 tbsp	14 g/½ oz	15	**107**	4.1	4
Flavoured milk, past. (*see also* milkshakes, below)	1 glass	200 ml/7 fl oz	128	**64**	1.5	4
Flavoured milk, pasteurized, chocolate	1 glass	200 ml/7 fl oz	123	**63**	1.5	4
Goats' milk, pasteurized	1 glass	200 ml/7 fl oz	124	**62**	3.7	5
Sheeps' milk, raw	1 glass	200 ml/7 fl oz	186	**93**	5.8	7
Soya milk, sweetened and calcium enriched	1 glass	200 ml/7 fl oz	86	**43**	2.4	4
Soya milk, unsweetened	1 glass	200 ml/7 fl oz	52	**26**	1.6	5
Buttermilk	2 tbsp	30 ml/1 fl oz	13	**44**	0.3	6

Milk Shakes

	Typical portion	Typical portion size	Calories per portion	Calories per 100 g/ml	Fat per 100 g/ml	Health rating (1–10)
Milk shake, thick	1 glass	200 ml/7 fl oz	176	**88**	1.8	2
Milk shake powder, made up with whole milk	1 glass	227 ml/8 fl oz	217	**87**	3.7	4
Milk shake powder, made up with s.-skim. milk	1 glass	227 ml/8 fl oz	172	**69**	1.6	5
Milk shake takeaway/fast food, large	1	432 ml/¾ pint	545	**126**	3.0	2
Milk shake takeaway/fast food medium	1	338 ml/11⅜ fl oz	425	**126**	3.0	2
Milk shake takeaway/fast food small	1	178 ml/6¼ fl oz	226	**126**	3.0	2

Milk products

	Typical portion	Typical portion size	Calories per portion	Calories per 100 g/ml	Fat per 100 g/ml	Health rating (1–10)
Crème caramel	1 pot	100 g/3½ oz	109	**109**	2.2	4
Custard, ready to eat	2 tbsp	56 g/2 oz	55	**98**	2.9	4
Custard, made up with whole milk	2 tbsp	56 g/2 oz	67	**118**	4.5	5
Custard, made up with semi-skimmed milk	2 tbsp	56 g/2 oz	54	**95**	2.0	5
Instant whipping dessert, banana flavour	2 tbsp	56 g/2 oz	274	**490**	21.0	3
Instant whipping dessert, butterscotch flavour	2 tbsp	56 g/2 oz	266	**475**	19.0	3

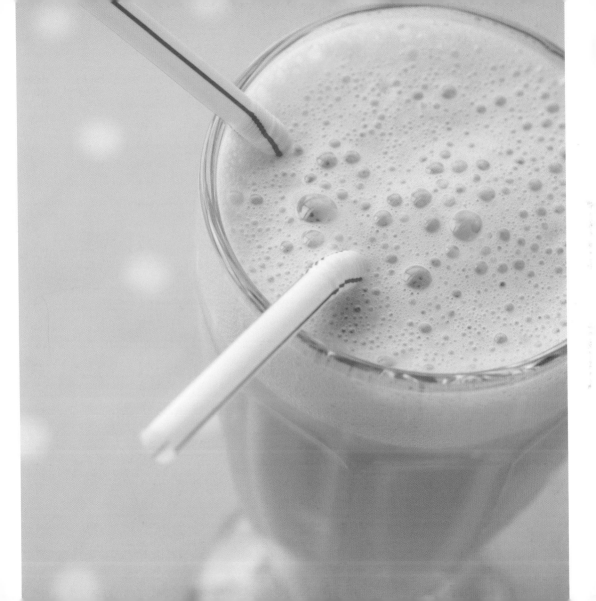

	Typical portion	Typical portion size	Calories per portion	Calories per 100 g/ml	Fat per 100 g/ml	Health rating (1–10)
Instant whipping dessert, chocolate flavour	2 tbsp	56 g/2 oz	252	**450**	22.0	3
Instant whipping dessert, forest fruit flavour	2 tbsp	56 g/2 oz	274	**490**	21.5	3
Instant whip. dess., raspberry/strawberry flavour	2 tbsp	56 g/2 oz	277	**495**	26.0	3
Instant dessert powder	2 tbsp	56 g/2 oz	218	**391**	17.3	3
Milk pudding, made with whole milk	1 pot	90 g/3¼ oz	117	**130**	4.3	4
Mousse, chocolate	1 pot	90 g/3¼ oz	134	**149**	6.5	3
Mousse, chocolate, reduced fat	1 pot	90 g/3¼ oz	111	**123**	3.7	4
Mousse, fruit	1 pot	90 g/3¼ oz	128	**143**	6.4	4
Panna cotta, caramel	1 pot	100 g/3½ oz	279	**279**	13.1	4
Panna cotta, strawberry	1 pot	100 g/3½ oz	100	**100**	2.6	4
Tzatziki	¼ pot	50 g/2 oz	63	**126**	10.6	5
Tzatziki, Greek authentic	¼ pot	50 g/2 oz	49	**99**	7.0	5

Fromage Frais

	Typical portion	Typical portion size	Calories per portion	Calories per 100 g/ml	Fat per 100 g/ml	Health rating (1–10)
Fromage frais, plain	2 tbsp	56 g/2 oz	64	**113**	8.0	6
Fromage frais, fruit	1 pot	100 g/3½ oz	124	**124**	5.6	5
Fromage frais, virtually fat free, natural	2 tbsp	56 g/2 oz	27	**49**	0.1	6
Fromage frais, virtually fat free, fruit	2 tbsp	56 g/2 oz	28	**50**	0.2	6
Fromage frais, apricot	1 pot	100 g/3½ oz	77	**77**	3.0	4
Fromage frais, apricot, low fat	1 pot	100 g/3½ oz	58	**58**	0.1	4
Fromage frais, black cherry	1 pot	100 g/3½ oz	113	**113**	5.0	3
Fromage frais, black cherry, low fat	1 pot	100 g/3½ oz	54	**54**	0.2	4
Fromage frais, cherry, 0% fat	1 pot	100 g/3½ oz	59	**59**	0.1	4

	Typical portion	Typical portion size	Calories per portion	Calories per 100 g/ml	Fat per 100 g/ml	Health rating (1–10)
Fromage frais, natural plain, fat free	1 pot	100 g/3½ oz	49	**49**	0.1	4
Fromage frais, strawberry, kids	1 pot	100 g/3½ oz	101	**101**	1.3	4
Fromage frais, toffee and pecan pie	1 pot	100 g/3½ oz	148	**148**	6.8	3
Yogurt						
Drinking yogurt (e.g. Yakult)	1 pot	33g/1⅙ oz	21	**62**	0.1	4
Greek-style yogurt, plain	2 tbsp	56 g/2 oz	75	**133**	10.2	6
Greek-style yogurt, fruit	1 pot	100 g/3½ oz	137	**137**	8.4	6
Greek yogurt, sheep	2 tbsp	56 g/2 oz	52	**92**	6.0	6
Lassi, sweetened	2 tbsp	56 g/2 oz	35	**62**	0.9	4
Low-fat yogurt, plain	2 tbsp	56 g/2 oz	32	**56**	1.0	6
Low-fat yogurt, fruit	1 pot	100 g/4 oz	78	**78**	1.1	6
Virtually fat free/diet yogurt, plain	2 tbsp	56 g/2 oz	31	**54**	0.2	5
Virtually fat free/diet yogurt, fruit	1 pot	100 g/4 oz	47	**47**	0.2	4
Whole milk yogurt, plain	2 tbsp	56 g/2 oz	45	**79**	3.0	6
Whole milk yogurt, fruit	1 pot	100 g/4 oz	109	**109**	3.0	5
Whole milk yogurt, infant, fruit	1 pot	50 g/2 oz	45	**90**	3.7	5
Cream						
Cream, single	1 tbsp	14 g/½ oz	27	**193**	19.1	2
Cream, sour	1 tbsp	14 g/½ oz	29	**205**	19.9	3
Cream, whipping	1 tbsp	14 g/½ oz	53	**381**	40.3	2
Cream, double	1 tbsp	14 g/½ oz	69	**496**	57.3	2
Cream, clotted	1 tbsp	14 g/½ oz	82	**586**	63.5	2

	Typical portion	Typical portion size	Calories per portion	Calories per 100 g/ml	Fat per 100 g/ml	Health rating (1–10)
Crème fraîche	1 tbsp	14 g/½ oz	53	**378**	40.0	4
Crème fraîche, half fat	1 tbsp	14 g/½ oz	23	**162**	15.0	5
Dairy cream, extra thick	1 tbsp	14 g/½ oz	33	**236**	23.5	2
Dairy cream, UHT canned, spray	1 dssp	8 g/¼ oz	20	**252**	24.2	2
Dairy cream, UHT canned, spray, half fat	1 dssp	8 g/¼ oz	16	**196**	17.3	3
Cream, sterilized, canned	1 tbsp	14 g/½ oz	33	**239**	23.9	2
Imitation cream (e.g. Elmlea), single	1 tbsp	14 g/½ oz	22	**158**	14.5	2
Imitation cream, single, whipping	1 tbsp	14 g/½ oz	41	**292**	29.9	2
Imitation cream, double	1 tbsp	14 g/½ oz	48	**345**	35.7	2
Dessert topping (e.g. Tip Top)	1 tbsp	14 g/½ oz	16	**112**	6.5	1

Ice Creams – *see* Snacks, Confectionery & Desserts, page 224

Butter and Spreads

	Typical portion	Typical portion size	Calories per portion	Calories per 100 g/ml	Fat per 100 g/ml	Health rating (1–10)
Butter	1 tsp	5 g/⅙ oz	37	**744**	82.2	3
Butter, spreadable	1 tsp	5 g/⅙ oz	38	**745**	82.5	3
Butter, blended spread (70–80% fat)	1 tsp	5 g/⅙ oz	34	**680**	74.8	3
Butter, blended spread (40% fat)	1 tsp	5 g/⅙ oz	20	**390**	40.3	3
Buttermilk-based spread/creamery	1 tsp	5 g/⅙ oz	37	**735**	81.3	3
Buttermilk-based spread/creamery, reduced fat	1 tsp	5 g/⅙ oz	19	**368**	39.4	3
Buttermilk-based spread/creamery, salted	1 tsp	5 g/⅙ oz	37	**729**	81.1	2
Dairy spread	1 tsp	5 g/⅙ oz	19	**388**	40.0	2
Margarine, hard, animal and vegetable fats	1 tsp	5 g/⅙ oz	36	**718**	79.3	2
Margarine, hard, vegetable fats only	1 tsp	5 g/⅙ oz	37	**742**	82.3	2

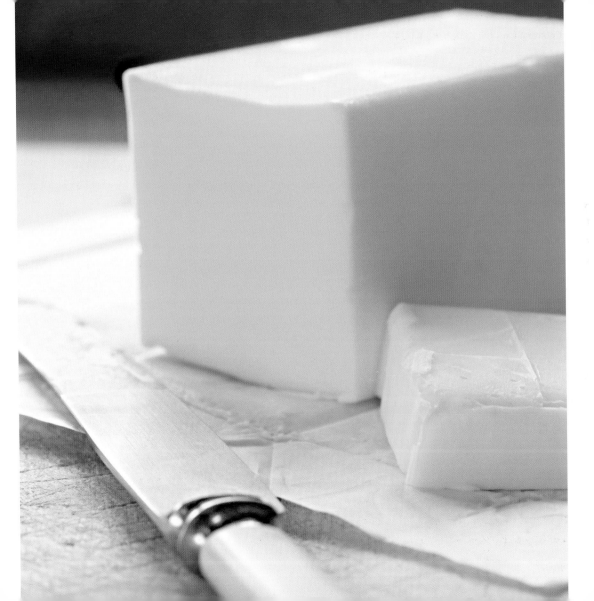

Counting Calories: Eggs, Dairy & Fats

	Typical portion	Typical portion size	Calories per portion	Calories per 100 g/ml	Fat per 100 g/ml	Health rating (1–10)
Margarine, soft, not polyunsaturated	1 tsp	5 g/⅙ oz	37	**740**	81.7	2
Margarine, soft, polyunsaturated	1 tsp	5 g/⅙ oz	37	**746**	82.8	1
Margarine, no salt	1 tsp	5 g/⅙ oz	27	**531**	59.0	1
Margarine, light	1 tsp	5 g/⅙ oz	15	**218**	23.0	1
Margarine, soya	1 tsp	5 g/⅙ oz	52	**745**	82.0	1
Margarine, white	1 tsp	5 g/⅙ oz	60	**855**	95.0	1
Fat spread (70-80% fat), not polyunsaturated	1 tsp	5 g/⅙ oz	32	**642**	71.2	1
Fat spread (40% fat), not polyunsaturated	1 tsp	5 g/⅙ oz	18	**368**	37.5	1
Fat spread (20-25% fat), not polyunsaturated	1 tsp	5 g/⅙ oz	13	**262**	25.5	1
Fat spread (70% fat), polyunsaturated	1 tsp	5 g/⅙ oz	31	**622**	68.5	2
Fat spread (60% fat), polyunsaturated	1 tsp	5 g/⅙ oz	27	**553**	60.8	2
Fat spread (35-40% fat), polyunsaturated	1 tsp	5 g/⅙ oz	19	**365**	37.6	3
Fat spread (20% fat), polyunsaturated	1 tsp	5 g/⅙ oz	9	**183**	20.0	3
Fat spread (5% fat)	1 tsp	5 g/⅙ oz	6	**115**	5.0	3
Fat spread (60% fat), with olive oil	1 tsp	5 g/⅙ oz	28	**569**	62.7	2
Garlic butter	1 tsp	5 g/⅙ oz	34	**686**	75.0	3

Fats and Oils

	Typical portion	Typical portion size	Calories per portion	Calories per 100 g/ml	Fat per 100 g/ml	Health rating (1–10)
Compound cooking fat	1 tsp	5 g/⅙ oz	45	**899**	99.9	1
Ghee, butter	1 tbsp	16 g/½ oz	144	**898**	99.8	1
Ghee, palm	1 tbsp	16 g/½ oz	144	**897**	99.7	1
Ghee, vegetable	1 tbsp	16 g/½ oz	143	**895**	99.4	1
Lard	1 tsp	5 g/⅙ oz	44	**891**	99.0	1

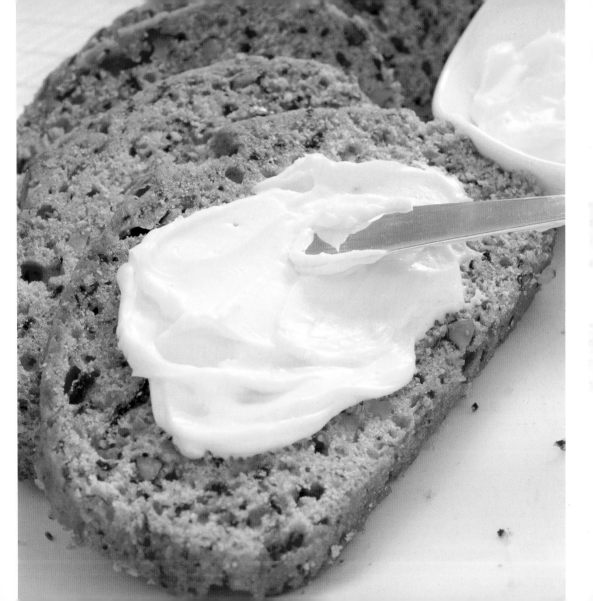

Counting Calories: Eggs, Dairy & Fats

	Typical portion	Typical portion size	Calories per portion	Calories per 100 g/ml	Fat per 100 g/ml	Health rating (1–10)
Suet, shredded	1 dssp	10 g/¼ oz	41	**826**	86.7	1
Suet, vegetable	1 dssp	10 g/¼ oz	41	**836**	87.9	1
Avocado oil	1 dssp	10 ml/⅓ fl oz	80	**802**	88.0	3
Chilli oil	1 dssp	10 ml/⅓ fl oz	83	**823**	91.5	2
Chinese stir-fry oil	1 dssp	10 ml/⅓ fl oz	83	**823**	91.4	2
Coconut oil	1 dssp	10 ml/⅓ fl oz	44	**899**	99.9	2
Cod liver oil	1 dssp	10 ml/⅓ fl oz	90	**899**	99.9	7
Corn oil	1 dssp	10 ml/⅓ fl oz	44	**899**	99.9	2
Evening primrose oil	1 tsp	5 ml/⅙ fl oz	44	**899**	99.9	7
Flaxseed oil	1 tsp	5 ml/⅙ fl oz	42	**829**	92.5	7
Grapeseed oil	1 tsp	5 ml/⅙ fl oz	43	**865**	96.1	4
Groundnut/peanut oil	1 tsp	5 ml/⅙ fl oz	41	**824**	91.8	4
Hazelnut oil	1 tsp	5 ml/⅙ fl oz	45	**899**	99.9	4
Linseed oil	1 tsp	5 ml/⅙ fl oz	42	**837**	93.0	7
Macadamia oil	1 tsp	5 ml/⅙ fl oz	40	**805**	91.0	4
Olive oil	1 dssp	10 ml/⅓ fl oz	90	**899**	99.9	5
Olive oil, extra virgin	1 dssp	10 ml/⅓ fl oz	90	**848**	94.5	6
Olive oil, extra virgin, 1-cal spray	1 dssp	10 ml/⅓ fl oz	50	**498**	55.2	5
Olive oil, mild	1 dssp	10 ml/⅓ fl oz	86	**861**	95.7	5
Palm oil	1 dssp	10 ml/⅓ fl oz	44	**899**	99.9	2
Rapeseed oil	1 dssp	10 ml/⅓ fl oz	44	**899**	99.9	4
Safflower oil	1 dssp	10 ml/⅓ fl oz	44	**899**	99.9	6

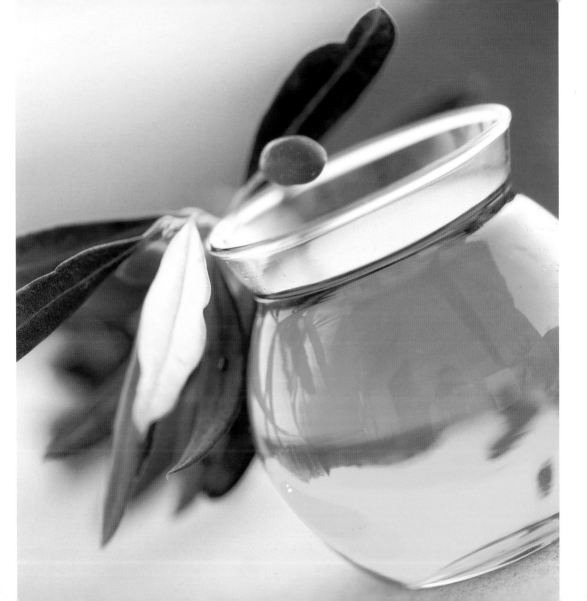

	Typical portion	Typical portion size	Calories per portion	Calories per 100 g/ml	Fat per 100 g/ml	Health rating (1–10)
Sesame oil	1 tsp	5 ml/⅙ fl oz	45	**892**	99.9	5
Soya oil	1 dssp	10 ml/⅓ fl oz	44	**899**	99.9	2
Sunflower oil	1 dssp	10 ml/⅓ fl oz	44	**899**	99.9	5
Vegetable oil, blended	1 dssp	10 ml/⅓ fl oz	44	**899**	99.9	3
Walnut oil	1 dssp	10 g/¼ oz	44	**899**	99.9	6
Wheatgerm oil	1 dssp	10 g/¼ oz	44	**899**	99.9	6

Cheeses

	Typical portion	Typical portion size	Calories per portion	Calories per 100 g/ml	Fat per 100 g/ml	Health rating (1–10)
Brie	1 wedge	50 g/2 oz	172	**343**	29.1	4
Camembert	1 wedge	50 g/2 oz	145	**290**	22.7	4
Cheddar, medium	1 wedge	50 g/2 oz	206	**411**	34.5	5
Cheddar type, half-fat	1 wedge	50 g/2 oz	137	**273**	15.8	5
Cheddar, vegetarian	1 wedge	50 g/2 oz	195	**390**	32.0	4
Cheese spread, plain	1 tbsp	40 g/1½ oz	107	**267**	22.8	2
Cheese spread, reduced fat	1 tbsp	40 g/1½ oz	70	**175**	9.5	3
Cottage cheese, plain	1 tbsp	40 g/1½ oz	41	**101**	4.3	6
Cottage cheese, plain, reduced fat	1 tbsp	40 g/1½ oz	28	**79**	1.5	6
Cottage cheese, plain, with additions	1 tbsp	40 g/1½ oz	38	**95**	3.8	5
Cream cheese	1 tbsp	40 g/1½ oz	176	**439**	47.4	3
Cream cheese, reduced fat	1 tbsp	40 g/1½ oz	47	**117**	5.3	4
Danish blue	1 wedge	50 g/2 oz	170	**342**	28.9	4
Dolcelatte	1 wedge	50 g/2 oz	183	**366**	32.3	4
Doux de Montagne	1 wedge	50 g/2 oz	176	**352**	28.3	4

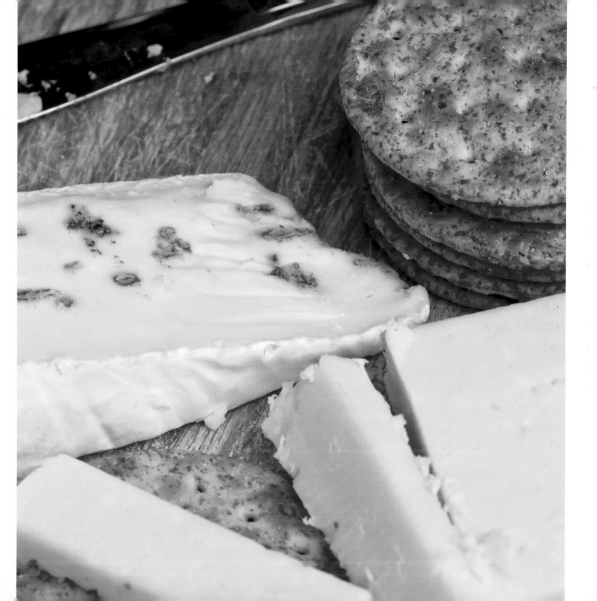

Counting Calories: Eggs, Dairy & Fats

	Typical portion	Typical portion size	Calories per portion	Calories per 100 g/ml	Fat per 100 g/ml	Health rating (1–10)
Edam	1 wedge	50 g/2 oz	171	**341**	26.0	5
Emmental	1 wedge	50 g/2 oz	184	**368**	28.3	5
Feta	1 wedge	50 g/2 oz	125	**250**	20.2	6
Goats' milk soft cheese, full fat with rind	1 wedge	50 g/2 oz	160	**320**	25.8	6
Gorgonzola	1 wedge	50 g/2 oz	167	**334**	27.0	5
Gouda	1 wedge	50 g/2 oz	189	**377**	30.6	5
Gruyère	1 wedge	50 g/2 oz	205	**409**	33.3	5
Halloumi	1 wedge	50 g/2 oz	158	**316**	24.7	5
Mascarpone	1 wedge	50 g/2 oz	219	**437**	4.1	5
Mozzarella, fresh	1 wedge	50 g/2 oz	129	**257**	20.3	5
Mozzarella, reduced fat	1 wedge	50 g/2 oz	129	**275**	1.2	6
Parmesan, fresh	1 wedge	50 g/2 oz	208	**415**	29.7	5
Processed cheese, plain (e.g. Dairylea)	1 triangle	17 g/⅗ oz	43	**250**	19.0	2
Processed cheese, slices, reduced fat	1 slice	17 g/⅗ oz	47	**275**	22.5	2
Ricotta	1 wedge	50 g/2 oz	67	**134**	9.5	4
Roquefort	1 wedge	50 g/2 oz	188	**375**	32.9	4
Roule	1 wedge	50 g/2 oz	161	**321**	30.5	3
Spreadable cheese, soft white, low fat	1 tbsp	40 g/1½ oz	53	**132**	8.0	2
Spreadable cheese, soft white, medium fat	1 tbsp	40 g/1½ oz	80	**199**	16.3	2
Spreadable cheese, soft white, full fat	1 tbsp	40 g/1½ oz	125	**312**	31.3	2
Stilton, blue	1 wedge	40 g/1½ oz	164	**410**	35.0	4
White cheese	1 wedge	40 g/1½ oz	152	**381**	31.8	5

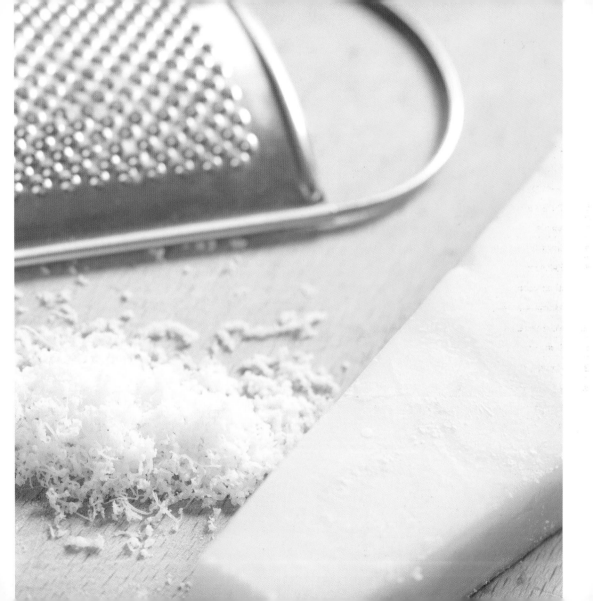

	Typical portion	Typical portion size	Calories per portion	Calories per 100 g/ml	Fat per 100 g/ml	Health rating (1–10)
Eggs and Egg Dishes						
Egg, chicken, whole, raw, large	1 egg	56 g/2 oz	80	**143**	9.9	7
Egg, chicken, whole, raw, medium	1 egg	50 g/2 oz	71	**143**	9.9	7
Egg, chicken, white, raw, large	1 egg	33 g/1⅙ oz	17	**52**	0.6	6
Egg, chicken, yolk, raw, large	1 egg	14 g/½ oz	47	**339**	30.5	7
Egg, chicken, boiled or poached, large	1 egg	56 g/2 oz	82	**147**	10.8	7
Egg, chicken, fried	1 egg	60 g/2 oz	107	**179**	13.9	4
Egg, chicken, scrambled, with milk, large	1 egg	56 g/2 oz	144	**257**	23.4	7
Egg, duck, whole, raw	1 egg	75 g/3 oz	122	**163**	11.8	7
Egg, goose, whole, raw	1 egg	144 g/5 oz	267	**185**	13.3	7
Egg, quail, whole, raw	1 egg	13 g/½ oz	20	**151**	11.1	7
Egg, turkey, whole, raw	1 egg	90 g/3¼ oz	149	**165**	12.2	7
Egg powder, white, dry	1 tbsp	14 g/½ oz	41	**295**	0.0	2
Egg powder, whole, dry	1 tbsp	14 g/½ oz	80	**568**	41.6	3
Omelette, plain, large	1 egg	56 g/2 oz	109	**195**	16.8	7
Omelette, cheese, large	2 eggs	105 g/3¾ oz	284	**271**	23.0	6
Omelette, ham and mushroom	1 omelette	120 g/4 oz	200	**167**	13.9	6
Omelette, mushroom and cheese	1 omelette	120 g/4 oz	248	**207**	17.9	6
Omelette, Spanish	1 omelette	120 g/4 oz	144	**120**	8.3	6
Quiche, cheese and egg	¼	82 g/3 oz	255	**315**	22.3	4
Quiche, cheese and egg, wholemeal	¼	82 g/3 oz	254	**309**	22.5	5
Quiche Lorraine	¼	82 g/3 oz	294	**358**	25.5	4

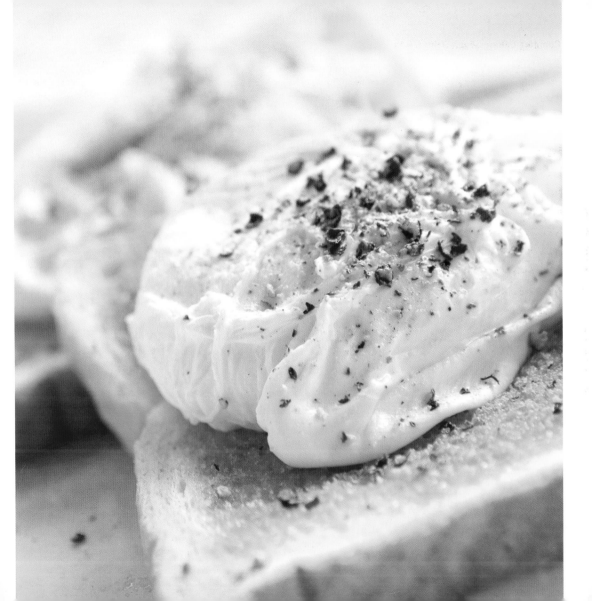

Grains, Cereals & Pastas

	Typical portion	Typical portion size	Calories per portion	Calories per 100 g/ml	Fat per 100 g/ml	Health rating (1–10)
Flour and Grains						
Besan flour	n/a	n/a	n/a	**313**	5.4	6
Bran	n/a	n/a	n/a	**206**	5.5	7
Bread flour, brown, strong	n/a	n/a	n/a	**311**	1.8	6
Bread flour, white, strong	n/a	n/a	n/a	**336**	1.5	7
Bread flour, wholemeal	n/a	n/a	n/a	**315**	2.2	8
Buckwheat	n/a	n/a	n/a	**364**	1.5	6
Bulgur wheat	n/a	n/a	n/a	**353**	1.7	6
Chapatti flour, white	n/a	n/a	n/a	**335**	0.5	4
Cornflour	n/a	n/a	n/a	**354**	0.7	4
Couscous, dry	3 tbsp	90 g/3¼ oz	320	**356**	1.5	5
Couscous, cooked	½ bag	200 g/7 oz	316	**158**	1.9	5
Chickpea flour	n/a	n/a	n/a	**313**	5.4	7
Millet flour	n/a	n/a	n/a	**354**	1.7	7
Oatmeal	n/a	n/a	n/a	**375**	9.2	8
Pearl barley, raw	n/a	n/a	n/a	**352**	1.2	5
Pearl barley, boiled	3 tbsp	80 g/3 oz	98	**123**	0.4	5
Polenta	2 tbsp	60 g/2 oz	214	**357**	1.4	5
Potato flour	n/a	n/a	n/a	**328**	0.9	7

	Typical portion	Typical portion size	Calories per portion	Calories per 100 g/ml	Fat per 100 g/ml	Health rating (1–10)
Quinoa grains, dry	n/a	n/a	n/a	**374**	5.8	6
Rice flour	n/a	n/a	n/a	**366**	0.8	7
Rye flour, wholemeal	n/a	n/a	n/a	**335**	2.0	8
Sago, raw	3 tbsp	80 g/3 oz	284	**355**	0.2	4
Soya flour, full fat	n/a	n/a	n/a	**447**	23.5	5
Soya flour, low fat	n/a	n/a	n/a	**352**	7.2	5
Spelt flour	n/a	n/a	n/a	**381**	2.9	7
Wheat flour, brown	n/a	n/a	n/a	**324**	2.0	7
Wheat flour, white, plain	n/a	n/a	n/a	**341**	1.3	4
Wheat flour, white self-raising	n/a	n/a	n/a	**330**	1.2	4
Wheat flour, wholemeal	n/a	n/a	n/a	**310**	2.2	7
Wheatgerm	n/a	n/a	n/a	**357**	9.2	8

Rice

	Typical portion	Typical portion size	Calories per portion	Calories per 100 g/ml	Fat per 100 g/ml	Health rating (1–10)
Arborio, dry	1 tbsp	50 g/2 oz	174	**348**	0.8	5
Basmati, brown, dry	1 tbsp	50 g/2 oz	176	**353**	3.0	6
Basmati, brown, cooked	½ bowl	140 g/5 oz	189	**135**	1.8	6
Basmati, Indian, dry	1 tbsp	50 g/2 oz	173	**346**	0.9	5
Basmati, white, dry	1 tbsp	50 g/2 oz	175	**349**	0.6	4
Basmati, wholegrain, cooked	½ bowl	140 g/5 oz	158	**113**	0.9	7
Brown, raw	1 tbsp	50 g/2 oz	179	**357**	2.8	6
Brown, boiled	½ bowl	140 g/5 oz	160	**141**	1.1	6
Long grain, American, dry	1 tbsp	50 g/2 oz	175	**350**	1.1	6

	Typical portion	Typical portion size	Calories per portion	Calories per 100 g/ml	Fat per 100 g/ml	Health rating (1–10)
Long grain, American, cooked	½ bowl	140 g/5 oz	73	**143**	1.7	5
Long grain, microwaveable, cooked	½ bowl	140 g/5 oz	168	**120**	0.6	5
Pilaf, plain	½ bowl	140 g/5 oz	199	**142**	4.6	5
White, easycook, raw	1 tbsp	50 g/2 oz	191	**383**	3.6	4
White, easycook, boiled	½ bowl	140 g/5 oz	193	**138**	1.3	4
White, fried	½ bowl	140 g/5 oz	201	**144**	4.1	2

Savoury Rice Dishes – *see also* Takeaway & Convenience Food, from page 238

	Typical portion	Typical portion size	Calories per portion	Calories per 100 g/ml	Fat per 100 g/ml	Health rating (1–10)
Kedgeree	6 tbsp	160 g/5½ oz	282	**176**	9.1	6
Paella, chicken, chorizo and king prawn	½ pack	200 g/7 oz	260	**130**	4.9	6
Paella, seafood	½ pack	200 g/7 oz	252	**126**	1.3	6
Pilaf, forest mushroom and pine nut	1 bowl	150 g/5 oz	225	**150**	6.5	6
Rice, chicken and sweetcorn	½ bowl	150 g/5 oz	488	**325**	2.8	6
Rice, coriander and herb	½ bowl	150 g/5 oz	554	**369**	3.5	5
Rice curry	½ bowl	150 g/5 oz	182	**121**	0.9	4
Rice, coconut and mushroom	½ bowl	150 g/5 oz	237	**158**	5.0	4
Rice and mixed vegetables	½ bowl	150 g/5 oz	563	**375**	2.7	6
Risotto, vegetable	1 bowl	225 g/8 oz	330	**147**	6.5	6
Risotto, beef	1 bowl	225 g/8 oz	778	**346**	5.9	6
Risotto, chicken and mushroom	1 bowl	225 g/8 oz	279	**124**	2.8	6
Risotto, caramelized onion and Gruyère cheese	1 bowl	225 g/8 oz	394	**175**	10.3	5
Risotto, smoked salmon and spinach	1 bowl	225 g/8 oz	315	**140**	8.0	6
Risotto, seafood	1 bowl	225 g/8 oz	272	**121**	3.7	6

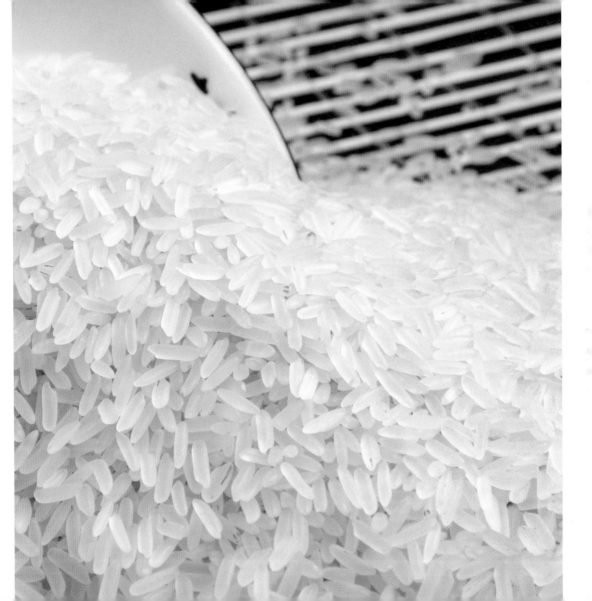

	Typical portion	Typical portion size	Calories per portion	Calories per 100 g/ml	Fat per 100 g/ml	Health rating (1–10)
Salad, rice and vegetables	1 bowl	150 g/5 oz	248	**165**	7.5	6
Savoury rice, raw	1 tbsp	40 g/1½ oz	166	**415**	10.3	4
Savoury rice, cooked	2 tbsp	90 g/3¼ oz	128	**142**	3.5	4
Pasta and Noodles						
Cannelloni tubes, dry	3 tubes	75 g/3 oz	270	**361**	3.6	4
Conchiglie shells, dry	3 tbsp	75 g/3 oz	258	**345**	1.5	4
Conchiglie shells, cooked	½ bowl	140 g/5 oz	186	**133**	0.8	4
Conchiglie shells, whole wheat, dry	3 tbsp	75 g/3 oz	237	**316**	2.0	4
Eliche, dry	3 tbsp	75 g/3 oz	264	**352**	1.9	4
Farfalle bows, dry	3 tbsp	75 g/3 oz	264	**353**	1.9	4
Fettucini, dry	3 tbsp	75 g/3 oz	271	**362**	1.7	4
Fusilli, dry	3 tbsp	75 g/3 oz	263	**351**	1.6	4
Fusilli, cooked	½ bowl	140 g/5 oz	165	**118**	0.6	4
Fusilli, fresh	½ bowl	140 g/5 oz	387	**277**	2.7	4
Fusilli, fresh, cooked	½ bowl	140 g/5 oz	230	**164**	1.8	4
Fusilli, wholemeal, dry	3 tbsp	75 g/3 oz	241	**322**	2.3	4
Garganelli, egg, dry	3 tbsp	75 g/3 oz	270	**360**	4.2	4
Lasagne sheets, dry	1 sheet	20 g/¾ oz	20	**100**	0.6	4
Lasagne sheets, fresh	1 sheet	20 g/¾ oz	54	**271**	2.1	4
Lasagne verdi sheets, dry	1 sheet	20 g/¾ oz	71	**355**	2.2	4
Macaroni, dry	3 tbsp	75 g/3 oz	265	**354**	1.7	4
Macaroni, raw	3 tbsp	75 g/3 oz	261	**348**	1.8	4

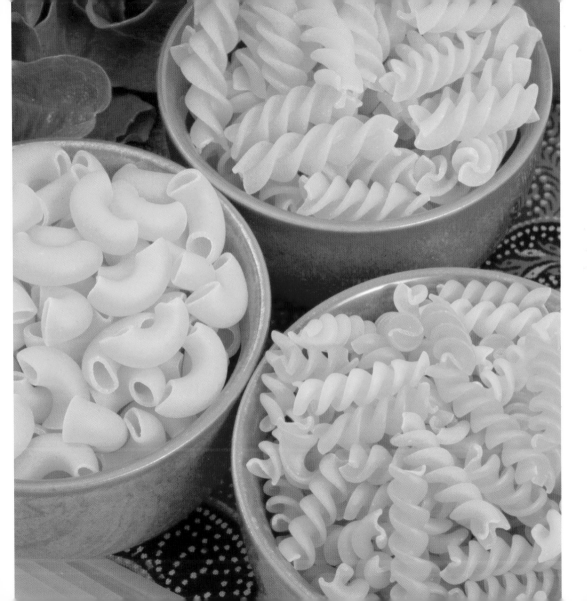

Counting Calories: Grains, Cereals & Pastas

	Typical portion	Typical portion size	Calories per portion	Calories per 100 g/ml	Fat per 100 g/ml	Health rating (1–10)
Macaroni, boiled	½ bowl	140 g/5 oz	121	**86**	0.5	4
Noodles, dry	1 handful	75 g/3 oz	225	**303**	0.4	4
Noodles, egg, dry	1 handful	75 g/3 oz	255	**340**	1.8	5
Noodles, boiled	½ bowl	140 g/5 oz	87	**62**	0.5	4
Noodles, fried	½ bowl	140 g/5 oz	146	**104**	5.3	2
Pappardelle, egg, dry	12 long strands	75 g/3 oz	273	**364**	3.7	5
Penne, dry	2 tbsp	75 g/3 oz	264	**352**	1.9	4
Penne, cooked	½ bowl	140 g/5 oz	185	**132**	0.7	4
Penne, fresh	½ bowl	140 g/5 oz	395	**282**	3.2	5
Penne, wholemeal, dry	2 tbsp	75 g/3 oz	243	**325**	2.5	7
Spaghetti etc. assorted, fresh, raw	12 long strands	75 g/3 oz	205	**274**	2.4	4
Spaghetti etc. assorted, fresh, cooked	½ bowl	140 g/5 oz	223	**159**	1.5	4
Spaghetti, white, raw	12 long strands	75 g/3 oz	256	**342**	1.8	4
Spaghetti, white, boiled	½ bowl	140 g/5 oz	146	**104**	0.7	4
Spaghetti, wholemeal, raw	12 long strands	75 g/3 oz	243	**324**	2.5	6
Spaghetti, wholemeal, boiled	½ bowl	140 g/5 oz	159	**113**	0.9	6
Tagliatelle, dry	12 long strands	75 g/3 oz	267	**356**	1.8	3
Tagliatelle, egg, dry	12 long strands	75 g/3 oz	271	**362**	3.3	4
Tagliatelle, fresh	12 long strands	75 g/3 oz	207	**276**	2.8	4
Tagliatelle verdi, fresh	½ bowl	140 g/5 oz	192	**137**	1.5	4
Trottole, dry	2 tbsp	75 g/3 oz	281	**375**	1.7	4

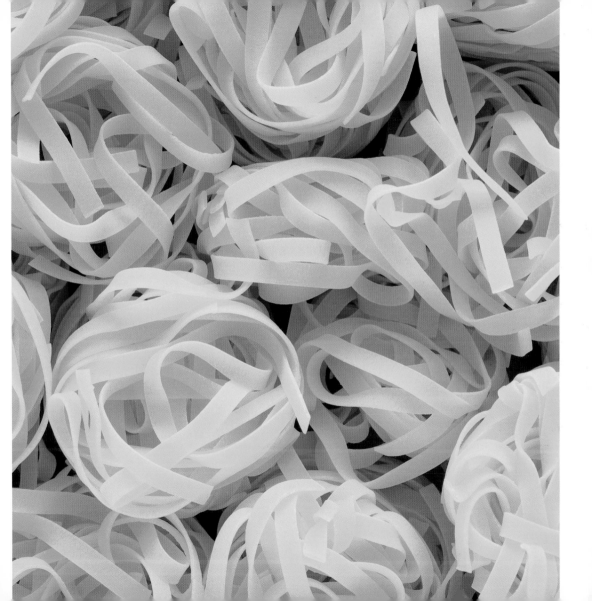

Counting Calories: Grains, Cereals & Pastas

	Typical portion	Typical portion size	Calories per portion	Calories per 100 g/ml	Fat per 100 g/ml	Health rating (1–10)
Pasta Dishes						
Cannelloni, beef	1 pack	300 g/11 oz	399	**133**	7.4	5
Cannelloni, beef and red wine	1 pack	300 g/11 oz	627	**209**	9.4	5
Cannelloni, chicken and pesto	1 pack	300 g/11 oz	450	**150**	7.5	6
Cannelloni, mediterranean vegetable	1 pack	300 g/11 oz	582	**194**	9.0	6
Cannelloni, mushroom	1 pack	300 g/11 oz	399	**133**	6.9	5
Cannelloni, pork	1 pack	300 g/11 oz	345	**115**	6.2	4
Cannelloni, ricotta and spinach	1 pack	300 g/11 oz	366	**122**	7.3	4
Cannelloni, smoked salmon	1 pack	300 g/11 oz	399	**133**	6.2	6
Cannelloni, spinach and wild mushroom	1 pack	300 g/11 oz	336	**112**	4.0	5
Cannelloni, vegetable	1 pack	300 g/11 oz	483	**161**	9.1	6
Cappelletti, goats' cheese and red pesto	½ pack	125 g/4 oz	374	**299**	8.7	5
Cappelletti and Italian meats	½ pack	125 g/4 oz	331	**265**	6.3	4
Cappelletti and Parma ham	½ pack	125 g/4 oz	367	**294**	9.2	4
Chicken alfredo	1 pack	200 g/7 oz	208	**104**	2.7	5
Fagottini, mushroom	½ pack	155 g/5½ oz	339	**219**	7.5	4
Fettucini, Cajun chicken, low fat range	6 tbsp	350 g/12 oz	396	**113**	2.2	5
Fettucini, chicken and mushroom, low fat range	6 tbsp	350 g/12 oz	315	**90**	1.7	5
Fettucini, tomatoes and mushroom	3 tbsp	175 g/6 oz	672	**384**	7.2	4
Lasagne, vegetable	3 tbsp	140 g/5 oz	164	**117**	5.3	4
Lasagne, beef	3 tbsp	150 g/5 oz	206	**137**	7.2	5
Lasagne, individual, chilled	1	225g/8 oz	430	**191**	10.8	4

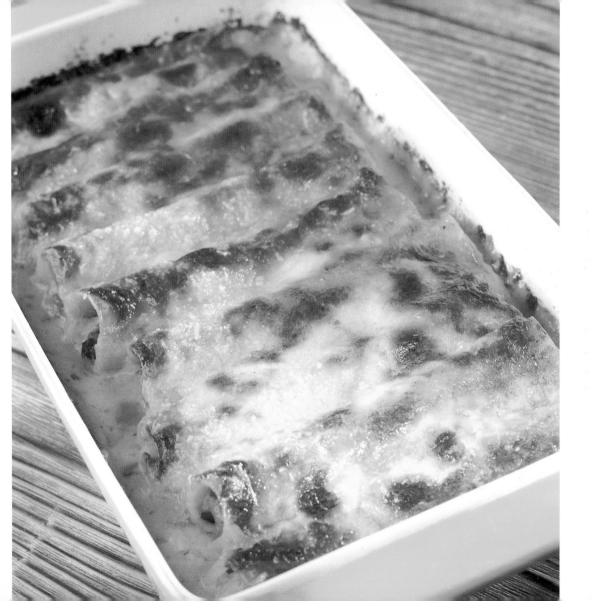

Counting Calories: Grains, Cereals & Pastas

	Typical portion	Typical portion size	Calories per portion	Calories per 100 g/ml	Fat per 100 g/ml	Health rating (1–10)
Lasagne, individual, frozen	1	225g/8 oz	321	**143**	6.1	4
Lasagne, bolognese and vegetable, diet	3 tbsp	140 g/5 oz	130	**93**	2.6	4
Lasagne, creamy ricotta and vegetable	3 tbsp	150 g/5 oz	159	**106**	2.8	4
Lasagne, vegetarian	½ pack	180 g/6⅓ oz	225	**125**	5.6	4
Macaroni cheese	6 tbsp	300 g/11 oz	534	**178**	10.8	3
Macaroni cheese, fresh	6 tbsp	300 g/11 oz	300	**100**	2.0	4
Macaroni cheese, canned	6 tbsp	300 g/11 oz	360	**120**	6.0	2
Noodles with chilli beef	½ pack	200 g/7 oz	184	**92**	1.4	5
Noodles with chicken chow mein	½ pack	200 g/7 oz	186	**93**	1.4	5
Noodles with hot and sour king prawns	½ pack	200 g/7 oz	130	**65**	1.4	5
Noodles with barbecue beef	½ pack	200 g/7 oz	252	**126**	4.8	5
Pasta bake, cheese and tomato	½ pack	200 g/7 oz	236	**118**	4.2	4
Pasta bake, chicken and mushroom	½ pack	200 g/7 oz	266	**133**	7.7	4
Pasta bake, pepperoni and ham	½ pack	200 g/7 oz	236	**118**	0.6	4
Pasta with meat and tomato sauce	1 bowl	300 g/11 oz	303	**101**	3.6	4
Ravioli, cheese and tomato, fresh	3 tbsp	125 g/4 oz	342	**274**	11.2	4
Ravioli, meat	3 tbsp	150 g/5 oz	261	**174**	4.2	5
Ravioli, smoked ham, bacon and tomato	3 tbsp	150 g/5 oz	363	**242**	7.7	4
Ravioli, vegetable in tomato sauce, diet	3 tbsp	140 g/5 oz	97	**69**	2.1	5
Ravioli, canned in tomato sauce	½ can	200 g/7 oz	140	**70**	2.2	3
Seafood pasta	1 bowl	125 g/4 oz	134	**110**	4.8	6
Spaghetti, canned in tomato sauce	½ can	200 g/7 oz	128	**64**	0.4	4

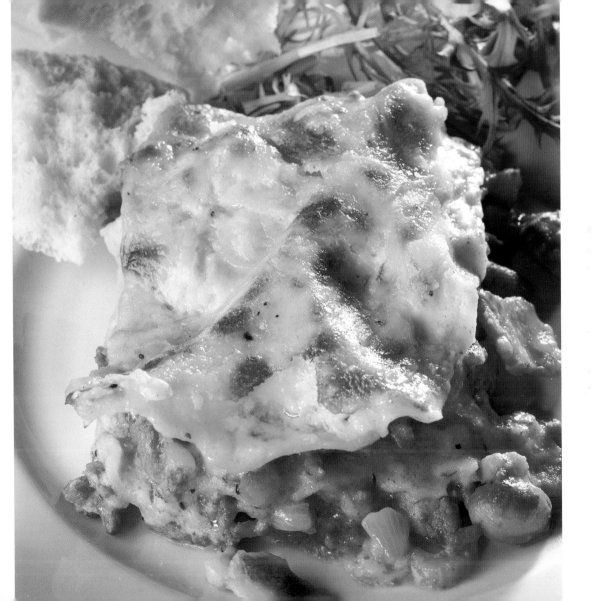

	Typical portion	Typical portion size	Calories per portion	Calories per 100 g/ml	Fat per 100 g/ml	Health rating (1–10)
Spaghetti bolognese, chilled/frozen, reheated	1 pack	225/8 oz	243	**108**	5.7	4
Spaghetti bolognese	1 pack	300 g/11 oz	318	**106**	2.9	4
Tagliatelle carbonara	6 tbsp	325 g/11½ oz	357	**102**	3.6	3
Tagliatelle, chicken and mushroom	6 tbsp	300 g/11 oz	270	**90**	1.7	5
Tagliatelle, ham and mushroom	6 tbsp	300 g/11 oz	360	**120**	5.1	4
Tagliatelle, salmon	6 tbsp	300 g/11 oz	282	**94**	2.7	5
Tagliatelle, vegetable	6 tbsp	300 g/11 oz	222	**74**	3.0	4
Tortellini, cheese and ham	3 tbsp	150 g/5 oz	396	**264**	8.2	3
Tortellini, beef bolognese	3 tbsp	150 g/5 oz	267	**178**	7.2	5
Tortellini, spinach and ricotta	3 tbsp	150 g/5 oz	382	**255**	4.2	4
Tortellini, tomato and mozzarella	3 tbsp	150 g/5 oz	236	**157**	2.8	3
Tortelloni, cheese and smoked ham	3 tbsp	150 g/5 oz	375	**250**	6.8	3
Tortelloni, five cheese	3 tbsp	150 g/5 oz	275	**183**	6.2	3
Tortelloni, olive and ricotta	3 tbsp	150 g/5 oz	345	**230**	10.5	3
Tortelloni, roasted vegetable	3 tbsp	150 g/5 oz	311	**207**	8.9	4

Breakfast Cereals

	Typical portion	Typical portion size	Calories per portion	Calories per 100 g/ml	Fat per 100 g/ml	Health rating (1–10)
All Bran-style cereal	½ bowl	45 g/1¾ oz	122	**270**	4.0	7
Bran flakes	½ bowl	45 g/1¾ oz	149	**330**	2.5	7
Bran flakes with sultanas	½ bowl	45 g/1¾ oz	142	**316**	2.0	6
Cheerios-style cereal	½ bowl	45 g/1¾ oz	166	**368**	3.8	5
Clusters (e.g. Nestlé-style)	½ bowl	45 g/1¾ oz	174	**387**	8.5	3
Cornflakes	½ bowl	45 g/1¾ oz	169	**376**	0.9	3

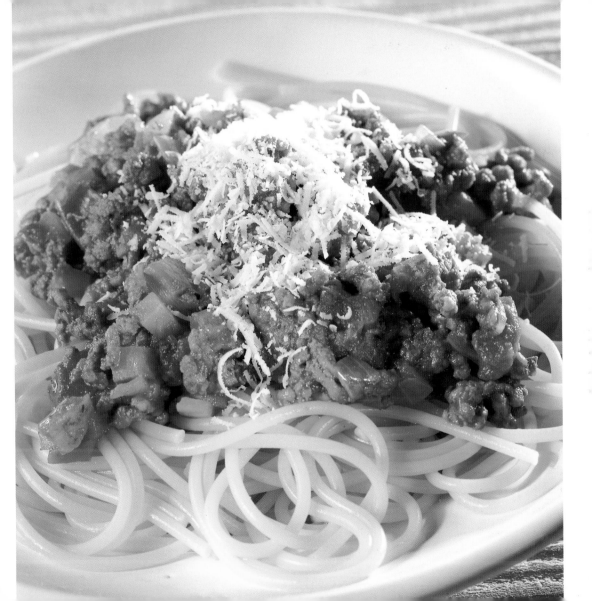

Counting Calories: Grains, Cereals & Pastas

	Typical portion	Typical portion size	Calories per portion	Calories per 100 g/ml	Fat per 100 g/ml	Health rating (1–10)
Cornflakes, honey-nut (e.g. Crunchy Nut)	½ bowl	45 g/1⅗ oz	182	**405**	3.5	2
Cornflakes, sugar-coated (e.g. Frosties)	½ bowl	45 g/1⅗ oz	171	**381**	0.6	2
Fruit and fibre flakes	½ bowl	45 g/1⅗ oz	159	**353**	5.0	5
Grits, old-fashioned	2 tbsp	41 g/1½ oz	38	**341**	1.2	4
Muesli, Swiss-style	½ bowl	45 g/1⅗ oz	163	**363**	5.9	4
Muesli, Swiss-style, no added sugar	½ bowl	45 g/1⅗ oz	165	**366**	7.8	5
Oat bran flakes	½ bowl	45 g/1⅗ oz	156	**346**	5.0	6
Porridge, instant (e.g. Ready Brek)	½ bowl	45 g/1⅗ oz	165	**366**	8.3	4
Porridge, made with water	½ bowl	45 g/1⅗ oz	20	**46**	1.1	6
Porridge, made with whole milk	½ bowl	45 g/1⅗ oz	51	**113**	5.1	7
Puffed wheat, sweetened (e.g. Sugar Puffs)	½ bowl	45 g/1⅗ oz	171	**381**	1.0	2
Puffed wheat, unsweetened	½ bowl	45 g/1⅗ oz	144	**321**	1.3	3
Rice and wheat flakes (e.g. Special K)	½ bowl	45 g/1⅗ oz	169	**376**	1.0	3
Shredded Wheat-style cereal	2 pieces	45 g/1⅗ oz	150	**332**	2.1	6
Toasted rice cereal, chocolate (e.g. Coco Pops)	½ bowl	45 g/1⅗ oz	172	**383**	2.5	3
Toasted rice cereal, plain (e.g. Rice Krispies)	½ bowl	45 g/1⅗ oz	172	**382**	1.0	3
Toasted rice cereal, sugar-coated (e.g. Ricicles)	½ bowl	45 g/1⅗ oz	170	**378**	4.0	3
Wholewheat biscuits (e.g. Weetabix)	2 biscuits	45 g/1⅗ oz	132	**352**	2.7	5
Wholewheat malted cereal (e.g. Shreddies)	½ bowl	45 g/1⅗ oz	156	**346**	1.9	5

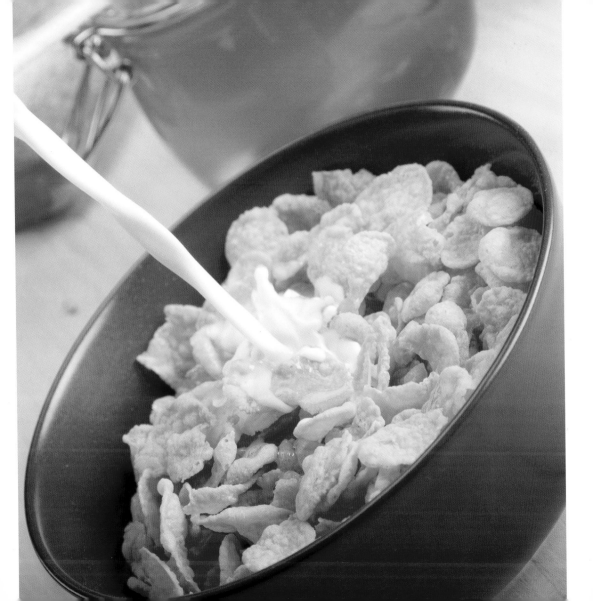

Nuts, Seeds & Pulses

	Typical portion	Typical portion size	Calories per portion	Calories per 100 g/ml	Fat per 100 g/ml	Health rating (1–10)
Beans and Pulses – *see also* Vegetables, page 118–19						
Aduki beans, cooked in unsalted water	1 tbsp	30 g/1 oz	37	**123**	0.2	7
Aduki beans, dried, raw	1 tbsp	30 g/1 oz	82	**272**	0.5	7
Baked beans, canned, in tomato sauce	½ can	207 g/7⅓ oz	155	**75**	0.2	4
Baked beans, as above, reduced sugar and salt	½ can	207 g/7⅓ oz	151	**73**	0.6	5
Baked beans and meatballs in tomato sauce	½ can	200 g/7 oz	216	**108**	3.6	3
Baked beans and jumbo sausages in tomato sauce	½ can	210/7⅓ oz	317	**151**	7	3
Baked beans and bacon	½ can	200 g/7 oz	182	**91**	1.7	3
Baked beans and chicken nuggets	½ can	200 g/7 oz	210	**105**	3.1	3
Baked beans and pork sausages	½ can	207 g/7⅓ oz	184	**89**	2.5	3
Baked beans and vegetable sausages	½ can	200 g/7 oz	212	**106**	3.6	3
Beansprouts, mung, raw	1 tbsp	30 g/1 oz	9	**31**	0.5	7
Beansprouts, mung, stir-fried in blended oil	3 tbsp	80 g/3 oz	22	**72**	6.1	4
Black beans, dried, raw	1 tbsp	30 g/1 oz	83	**275**	1.4	7
Black beans, boiled in salted water	3 tbsp	80 g/3 oz	72	**89**	0.4	7
Black-eye beans, dried, raw	1 tbsp	30 g/1 oz	93	**311**	1.6	7
Black-eye beans, boiled in unsalted water	3 tbsp	80 g/3 oz	92	**116**	0.7	7
Borlotti beans, dried, raw	1 tbsp	30 g/1 oz	100	**335**	1.2	7
Borlotti beans, canned	3 tbsp	80 g/3 oz	81	**103**	0.5	7

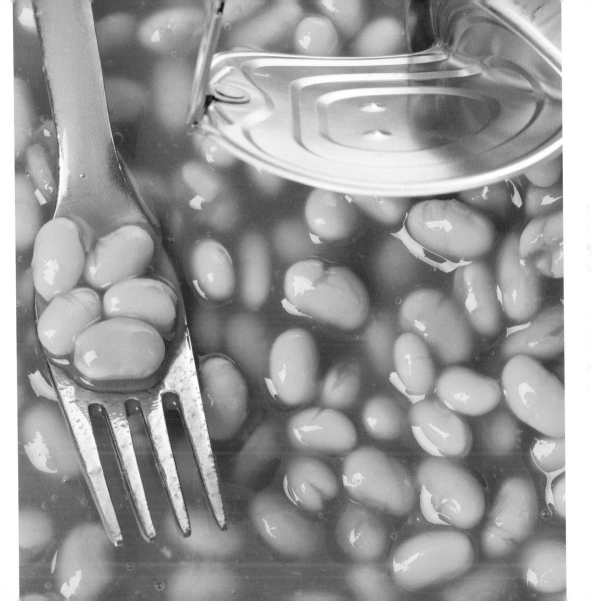

Counting Calories: Nuts, Seeds & Pulses

	Typical portion	Typical portion size	Calories per portion	Calories per 100 g/ml	Fat per 100 g/ml	Health rating (1–10)
Butter beans, canned	3 tbsp	80 g/3 oz	63	**79**	0.5	7
Butter beans, dried, boiled	3 tbsp	80 g/3 oz	85	**106**	0.6	7
Butter beans, dried, raw	1 tbsp	30 g/1 oz	87	**290**	1.7	7
Butter beans, in vegetable oil	3 tbsp	80 g/3 oz	91	**113**	4.6	4
Canellini beans	3 tbsp	80 g/3 oz	70	**87**	0.3	7
Canellini beans, curried	3 tbsp	80 g/3 oz	81	**103**	1.3	4
Chickpeas, whole, dried, raw	1 tbsp	30 g/1 oz	96	**320**	5.4	7
Chickpeas, whole, dried, boiled in unsalted water	3 tbsp	80 g/3 oz	97	**121**	2.1	7
Chickpeas, canned, reheated, drained	½ can	120 g/4 oz	138	**115**	2.9	7
Chilli beans, *see* Kidney beans, red, in chilli sauce						
Flageolet beans, canned	3 tbsp	80 g/3 oz	79	**99**	0.5	7
Haricot beans, dried, raw	1 tbsp	30 g/1 oz	86	**286**	1.6	7
Haricot beans, boiled in unsalted water	3 tbsp	80 g/3 oz	76	**95**	0.5	7
Kidney beans, red, raw	1 tbsp	30 g/1 oz	33	**266**	1.4	7
Kidney beans, red, boiled in unsalted water	3 tbsp	80 g/3 oz	82	**103**	0.5	7
Kidney beans, red, canned	½ can	120 g/4 oz	125	**104**	0.6	7
Kidney beans, red, in chilli sauce	3 tbsp	80 g/3 oz	73	**91**	0.7	7
Lentils, green and brown, whole, dried, raw	1 tbsp	30 g/1 oz	90	**297**	1.9	7
Lentils, as above, boiled in unsalted water	3 tbsp	80 g/3 oz	85	**105**	0.7	7
Lentils, red, split, dried, raw	1 tbsp	30 g/1 oz	96	**318**	1.3	7
Lentils, red, split, dried, boiled in unsalted water	3 tbsp	80 g/3 oz	80	**100**	0.4	7
Mixed beans, canned	½ can	150 g/5 oz	150	**100**	1.2	7

	Typical portion	Typical portion size	Calories per portion	Calories per 100 g/ml	Fat per 100 g/ml	Health rating (1–10)
Mixed beans, in hot spicy sauce	½ can	208 g/7⅓ oz	162	**78**	0.5	4
Mixed beans, in tomato sauce	½ can	210 g/7⅓ oz	242	**115**	0.1	6
Mung beans, whole, dried, raw	1 tbsp	30 g/1 oz	83	**279**	1.1	7
Mung beans, whole, dried, boiled in unsalted water	3 tbsp	80 g/3 oz	81	**91**	0.4	7
Pinto beans, dried, boiled in salted water	3 tbsp	80 g/3 oz	110	**137**	0.7	7
Pinto beans, dried, raw	1 tbsp	30 g/1 oz	98	**327**	1.6	7
Soya beans, dried, raw	1 tbsp	30 g/1 oz	98	**327**	1.6	7
Soya beans, dried, boiled in unsalted water	3 tbsp	80 g/3 oz	113	**141**	7.3	7
Tofu, soya bean, steamed	3 tbsp	80 g/3 oz	59	**73**	4.2	6
Tofu, soya bean, steamed, fried	3 tbsp	80 g/3 oz	208	**261**	17.7	3

Nuts and Seeds

	Typical portion	Typical portion size	Calories per portion	Calories per 100 g/ml	Fat per 100 g/ml	Health rating (1–10)
Almonds	1 handful	30 g/1 oz	184	**612**	54.8	7
Almonds, flaked	1 handful	30 g/1 oz	184	**613**	54.3	6
Almonds, toasted	1 handful	30 g/1 oz	190	**634**	56.4	7
Almonds, organic, shelled	1 handful	30 g/1 oz	189	**630**	55.8	7
Brazil nuts	1 handful	30 g/1 oz	205	**682**	68.2	7
Caraway seeds	1 pack	38 g/1⅓ oz	170	**448**	21.2	5
Cardamom seeds, black, ground	1 tsp	2 g/²⁄₂₈ oz	6	**311**	6.7	5
Cashew nuts, plain	1 handful	30 g/1 oz	175	**584**	48.9	6
Cashew nuts, roasted and salted	1 handful	30 g/1 oz	183	**611**	50.9	3
Chestnuts	1 handful	30 g/1 oz	51	**170**	2.7	9
Coconut, creamed block	n/a	n/a	n/a	**669**	68.8	3

Counting Calories: Nuts, Seeds & Pulses

	Typical portion	Typical portion size	Calories per portion	Calories per 100 g/ml	Fat per 100 g/ml	Health rating (1–10)
Coconut, desiccated	n/a	n/a	n/a	**604**	62	3
Coconut, fresh, flesh only	1 handful	50 g/2 oz	175	**351**	36	6
Coconut milk	½ can	200 ml/7 fl oz	348	**174**	17.4	3
Coconut milk, reduced fat	½ can	200 ml/7 fl oz	206	**103**	10	4
Fenugreek seeds	1 handful	30 g/1 oz	96	**323**	6.4	6
Flaxseed, milled	2 dssp	30 g/1 oz	153	**510**	46.2	8
Hazelnuts	1 handful	30 g/1 oz	195	**650**	63.5	7
Linseeds	1 tsp	5 g/⅙ oz	23	**464**	33.5	8
Macadamia nuts, salted	1 handful	30 g/1 oz	225	**748**	77.6	6
Melon seeds	1 handful	30 g/1 oz	174	**583**	47.7	6
Mixed nuts, chopped	1 handful	30 g/1 oz	180	**605**	50.9	6
Mixed nuts, unsalted	1 handful	30 g/1 oz	187	**622**	57.7	6
Mixed nuts, roasted	1 handful	30 g/1 oz	199	**662**	64	5
Mixed nuts, roasted, salted	1 handful	30 g/1 oz	188	**626**	58.4	4
Mixed nuts, honey roasted	1 handful	30 g/1 oz	175	**583**	45	3
Monkey nuts (peanuts in shells)	1 handful	50 g/2 oz	282	**565**	47.9	5
Mustard seeds	1 tsp	5 g/⅙ oz	23	**469**	28.8	5
Nigella seeds	1 tsp	5 g/⅙ oz	19	**392**	33.3	5
Peanuts and raisins	1 handful	30 g/1 oz	131	**435**	25.9	5
Peanuts, plain	1 handful	30 g/1 oz	169	**563**	46	5
Peanuts, dry roasted	1 handful	30 g/1 oz	177	**589**	49.8	2
Peanuts, roasted and salted	1 handful	30 g/1 oz	181	**602**	53	2

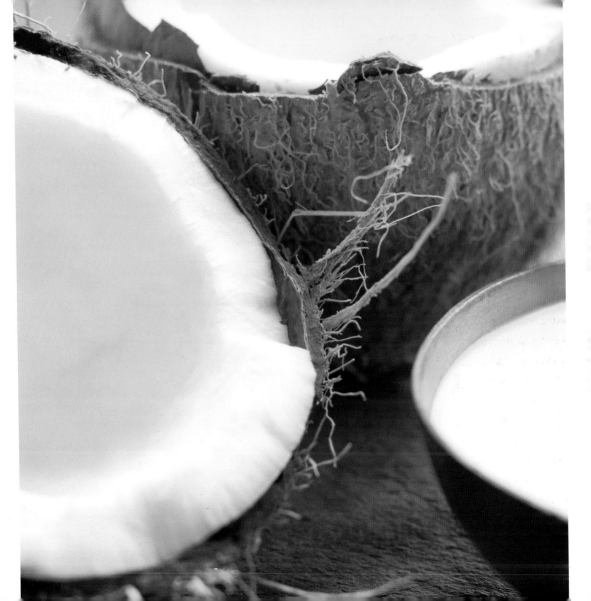

	Typical portion	Typical portion size	Calories per portion	Calories per 100 g/ml	Fat per 100 g/ml	Health rating (1–10)
Pecan nuts	1 handful	30 g/1 oz	206	**689**	70.1	7
Pine nuts	1 handful	30 g/1 oz	206	**688**	68.6	7
Pistachio nuts	1 handful	30 g/1 oz	180	**601**	55.4	6
Poppy seeds	1 tsp	5 g/⅙ oz	27	**533**	44.7	6
Pumpkin seeds	1 handful	30 g/1 oz	170	**568**	45.9	8
Pumpkin seeds, whole, roasted	1 handful	30 g/1 oz	156	**522**	42.1	8
Sesame seeds	1 handful	30 g/1 oz	183	**610**	56.4	7
Sunflower seeds	1 handful	30 g/1 oz	174	**585**	48.7	8
Trail mix	1 handful	30 g/1 oz	130	**432**	28.5	6
Walnuts	1 handful	30 g/1 oz	206	**688**	68.5	7

Nut, Seed and Pulse Products

	Typical portion	Typical portion size	Calories per portion	Calories per 100 g/ml	Fat per 100 g/ml	Health rating (1–10)
Carob powder	1 tbsp	2 g/²⁄₂₈ oz	3	**159**	0.1	6
Houmous	1 dssp	10 g/¼ oz	19	**187**	12.6	5
Marzipan, home-made	n/a	n/a	n/a	**462**	25.8	4
Marzipan, retail	n/a	n/a	n/a	**389**	12.7	3
Peanut butter, smooth	1 tsp	20 g/¾ oz	121	**606**	51.8	3
Peanut butter, crunchy	1 tsp	20 g/¾ oz	118	**592**	50.2	5
Peanut butter, whole-nut organic	1 tsp	20 g/¾ oz	122	**612**	48.7	6
Peanut butter, smooth, 33% less fat	1 tsp	20 g/¾ oz	107	**533**	35.1	4
Tahini paste	1 tbsp	30 g/1 oz	180	**607**	58.9	5

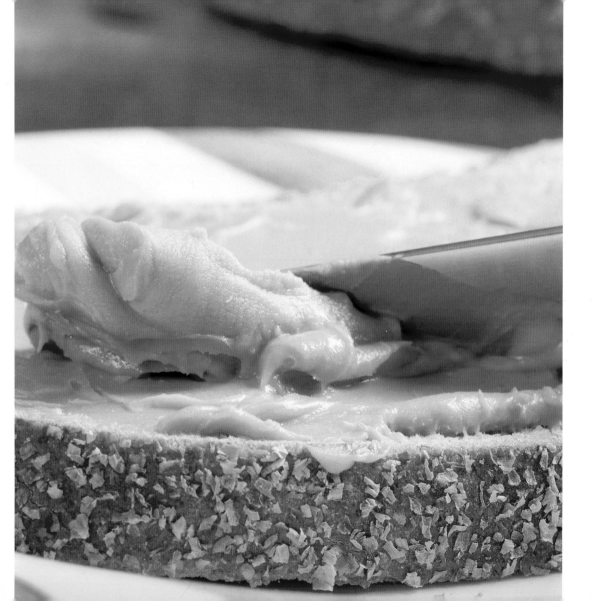

Meat & Poultry

	Typical portion	Typical portion size	Calories per portion	Calories per 100 g/ml	Fat per 100 g/ml	Health rating (1–10)
Beef						
Bison, raw	1 steak	140 g/5 oz	152	**109**	1.8	6
Bison, roasted	1 steak	100 g/3½ oz	143	**143**	2.4	6
Brisket, lean and fat, raw	3 tbsp	100 g/3½ oz	218	**218**	16.0	6
Brisket, lean, raw	3 tbsp	100 g/3½ oz	139	**139**	6.1	6
Dripping	1 tbsp	14 g/½ oz	125	**891**	99.0	1
Fat, cooked	1 tbsp	14 g/½ oz	75	**533**	52.3	1
Flank, lean and fat, pot-roasted	3 tbsp	100 g/3½ oz	309	**309**	22.3	6
Flank, lean, pot-roasted	3 tbsp	100 g/3½ oz	253	**253**	14.0	6
Forerib/rib-roast, lean and fat, raw	2 slices	120 g/4 oz	304	**253**	19.8	6
Forerib/rib-roast, lean and fat, roasted	2 slices	120 g/4 oz	360	**300**	20.4	6
Joint, sirloin, lean and fat, roasted	2 slices	140 g/5 oz	326	**233**	12.6	6
Joint, sirloin, lean, roasted	2 slices	140 g/5 oz	263	**188**	6.5	6
Mince, extra lean, raw	¼ pack	100 g/3½ oz	131	**131**	5.3	5
Mince, extra lean, stewed	¼ pack	100 g/3½ oz	177	**177**	8.7	6
Mince, lean, raw	¼ pack	100 g/3½ oz	175	**175**	9.7	5
Mince, raw	¼ pack	100 g/3½ oz	225	**225**	16.2	4
Mince, stewed	¼ pack	100 g/3½ oz	209	**209**	13.5	5
Ribeye steak	1 steak	340 g/12 oz	592	**174**	7.2	6

	Typical portion	Typical portion size	Calories per portion	Calories per 100 g/ml	Fat per 100 g/ml	Health rating (1–10)
Silverside, salted, boiled, lean	2 slices	140 g/5 oz	258	**184**	6.9	4
Steak, braising, lean and fat	¼ pack	100 g/3½ oz	246	**246**	12.7	6
Steak, braising, lean, braised	¼ pack	100 g/3½ oz	225	**225**	9.7	6
Steak, rump, from steakhouse, lean	1 large	342 g/12 oz	554	**162**	4.7	5
Steak, rump, lean and fat, fried	1 medium	228 g/8 oz	520	**228**	12.7	3
Steak, rump, lean and fat, raw	1 medium	228 g/8 oz	397	**174**	10.1	6
Steak, rump, lean, fried	1 medium	228 g/8 oz	417	**183**	6.6	3
Steak, rump, lean, grilled	1 medium	228 g/8 oz	404	**177**	5.9	6
Steak, rump, lean, raw	1 medium	228 g/8 oz	285	**125**	4.1	6
Steak, rump, strips, stir-fried, lean	¼ pack	140 g/5 oz	262	**208**	8.8	6
Steak, stewing, lean and fat, raw	¼ pack	140 g/5 oz	204	**146**	6.4	6
Steak, stewing, lean and fat, stewed	¼ pack	140 g/5 oz	284	**203**	9.6	6
Stir-fry strips, lean	¼ pack	100 g/3½ oz	104	**104**	2.0	6
Topside, lean and fat, raw	2 slices	140 g/5 oz	277	**198**	12.9	6
Topside, lean, roasted, well done	2 slices	140 g/5 oz	283	**202**	6.3	6
Topside, roasted, cold, thin sliced	2 slices	50 g/2 oz	52	**104**	2.5	6
Veal mince, raw	¼ pack	140 g/5 oz	202	**144**	7.0	5
Veal escalope, fried	1 escalope	120 g/4 oz	122	**196**	6.8	3
Veal, sirloin, lean and fat, roasted	2 slices	140 g/5 oz	283	**202**	10.4	5
Veal, sirloin, lean, roasted	2 slices	140 g/5 oz	235	**168**	6.2	5
Veal shoulder, lean and fat, roasted	2 slices	140 g/5 oz	256	**183**	8.2	5
Veal shoulder, lean, roasted	2 slices	140 g/5 oz	230	**164**	5.8	5

	Typical portion	Typical portion size	Calories per portion	Calories per 100 g/ml	Fat per 100 g/ml	Health rating (1–10)
Veal medallions	4 medallions	140 g/5 oz	228	**163**	2.5	5

Lamb

	Typical portion	Typical portion size	Calories per portion	Calories per 100 g/ml	Fat per 100 g/ml	Health rating (1–10)
Fat, cooked	1 tbsp	14 g/½ oz	80	**568**	56.3	1
Best-end neck cutlets, lean and fat, raw	1 cutlet	140 g/5 oz	442	**316**	27.9	6
Best-end neck cutlets, lean and fat, grilled	1 cutlet	120 g/4 oz	440	**367**	29.9	6
Best-end neck cutlets, lean, grilled	1 cutlet	120 g/4 oz	285	**238**	13.8	6
Breast, lean, roasted	2 slices	140 g/5 oz	382	**273**	18.5	6
Breast, lean and fat, roasted	2 slices	140 g/5 oz	503	**359**	29.9	6
Leg, lean and fat, raw	2 slices	140 g/5 oz	262	**187**	12.3	6
Leg, lean and fat, medium-roasted	2 slices	140 g/5 oz	336	**240**	14.2	6
Leg, lean, medium-roasted	2 slices	140 g/5 oz	284	**203**	9.4	6
Loin chops, lean and fat, raw	1 chop	140 g/5 oz	388	**277**	23.0	6
Loin chops, lean and fat, grilled	1 chop	120 g/4 oz	366	**305**	22.1	6
Loin chops, lean and fat, microwaved	1 chop	140 g/5 oz	493	**352**	26.9	5
Loin chops, lean and fat, roasted	1 chop	140 g/5 oz	503	**359**	26.9	6
Loin chops, lean, grilled	1 chop	120 g/4 oz	255	**213**	10.7	6
Mince, raw	¼ pack	140 g/5 oz	274	**196**	13.3	5
Mince, stewed	¼ pack	140 g/5 oz	291	**208**	12.3	5
Neck fillet, strips, lean, stir-fried	¼ pack	120 g/4 oz	334	**278**	20.0	5
Shoulder, lean and fat, raw	2 slices	140 g/5 oz	329	**235**	18.3	5
Shoulder, diced, lean and fat, grilled	¼ pack	120 g/4 oz	345	**288**	19.3	6
Shoulder, lean and fat, roasted	2 slices	140 g/5 oz	417	**298**	22.1	6

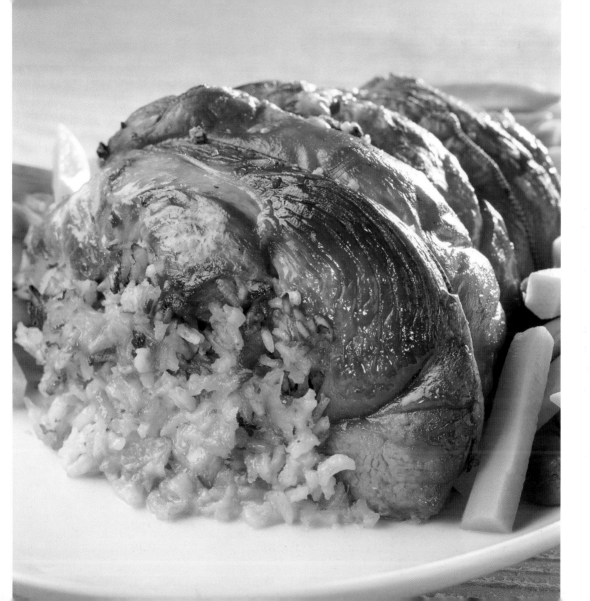

	Typical portion	Typical portion size	Calories per portion	Calories per 100 g/ml	Fat per 100 g/ml	Health rating (1–10)
Shoulder, lean, roasted	2 slices	140 g/5 oz	305	**218**	12.1	6
Stewing, lean, pressure-cooked	¼ pack	140 g/5 oz	347	**248**	14.8	6
Stewing, lean, stewed	¼ pack	140 g/5 oz	336	**240**	14.8	6
Stewing, lean and fat, stewed	¼ pack	140 g/5 oz	391	**279**	20.1	6
Goat						
Raw	1 steak	140 g/5 oz	153	**109**	2.3	6
Pork						
Bacon, back, raw	1 rasher	50 g/2 oz	107	**215**	16.5	4
Bacon, back, thick, raw	1 rasher	80 g/3 oz	172	**215**	16.5	4
Bacon, back, dry-fried	1 rasher	50 g/2 oz	148	**295**	22.0	3
Bacon, back, grilled	1 rasher	40 g/1½ oz	115	**287**	21.6	4
Bacon, back, grilled, crispy	1 rasher	35 g/1¼ oz	110	**313**	18.8	4
Bacon, back, microwaved	1 rasher	40 g/1⅜ oz	123	**307**	23.3	3
Bacon, back, fat trimmed, raw	1 rasher	50 g/2 oz	68	**136**	6.7	5
Bacon, back, fat trimmed, grilled	1 rasher	40 g/1½ oz	86	**214**	12.3	5
Bacon, back, reduced salt, grilled	1 rasher	40 g/1½ oz	113	**282**	20.6	5
Bacon, back, unsmoked, rindless, grilled	1 rasher	40 g/1½ oz	114	**284**	20.0	5
Bacon, back, smoked, grilled	1 rasher	40 g/1½ oz	117	**293**	22.1	4
Bacon, back, smoked, maple-cured, grilled	1 rasher	40 g/1½ oz	90	**225**	14.0	3
Bacon, back, sweet-cured, grilled	1 rasher	40 g/1½ oz	140	**351**	5.3	3
Bacon chops	1 chop	140 g/5 oz	315	**225**	18.0	5
Bacon chops, barbecued	1 chop	140 g/5 oz	330	**236**	14.8	4

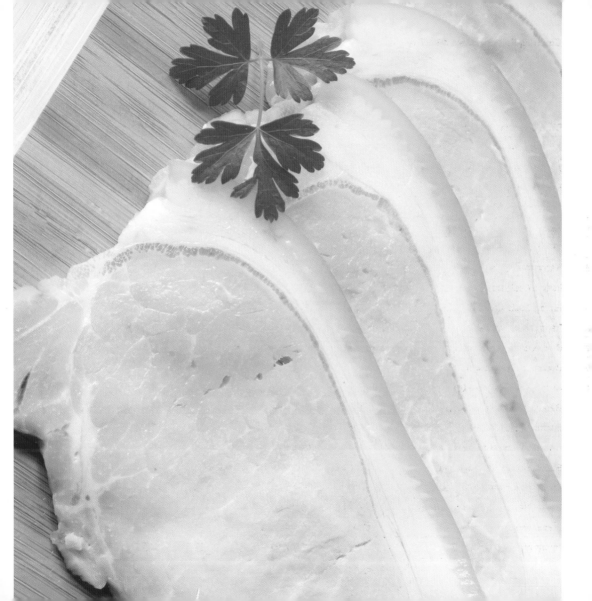

Counting Calories: Meat & Poultry

	Typical portion	Typical portion size	Calories per portion	Calories per 100 g/ml	Fat per 100 g/ml	Health rating (1–10)
Bacon chops, smoked	1 chop	140 g/5 oz	279	**199**	9.4	5
Bacon collar joint, lean and fat, raw	2 slices	140 g/5 oz	447	**319**	28.9	5
Bacon collar joint, lean and fat, boiled	2 slices	140 g/5 oz	455	**325**	27.0	5
Bacon collar joint, lean only, boiled	2 slices	140 g/5 oz	267	**191**	9.7	5
Bacon, fat only, raw	1 tbsp	13 g/½ oz	97	**747**	80.9	1
Bacon, fat only, cooked	1 tbsp	14 g/½ oz	97	**692**	72.8	1
Bacon, gammon rasher, lean only, grilled	2 slices	140 g/5 oz	241	**172**	5.2	5
Bacon, gammon rasher, lean only, fried	2 slices	140 g/5 oz	465	**332**	22.3	3
Bacon loin steak, grilled	1 steak	120 g/4 oz	229	**191**	9.7	5
Bacon, middle, raw	1 rasher	40 g/1½ oz	97	**241**	20.0	4
Bacon, middle, grilled	1 rasher	40 g/1½ oz	123	**307**	23.1	4
Bacon, middle, fried	1 rasher	40 g/1½ oz	140	**350**	28.5	3
Bacon, streaky, raw	1 rasher	40 g/1½ oz	110	**276**	23.6	4
Bacon, streaky, grilled	1 rasher	35 g/1¼ oz	118	**337**	26.9	4
Bacon, streaky, fried	1 rasher	40 g/1½ oz	134	**335**	26.6	3
Bacon, vegetarian	1 rasher	20 g/¾ oz	41	**203**	11.1	3
Bacon, vegetarian, streaky-style	1 rasher	8 g/¼ oz	17	**215**	10.6	3
Ham, baked	2 slices	140 g/5 oz	200	**143**	5.8	5
Ham, breaded	1 slice	37 g/1⅓ oz	57	**155**	6.3	4
Ham, breaded, dry-cured	1 slice	33 g/1⅙ oz	47	**142**	5.4	4
Ham, gammon joint, raw	2 slices	120 g/4¼ oz	166	**138**	7.5	5
Ham, gammon joint, boiled	2 slices	120 g/4¼ oz	245	**204**	12.3	5

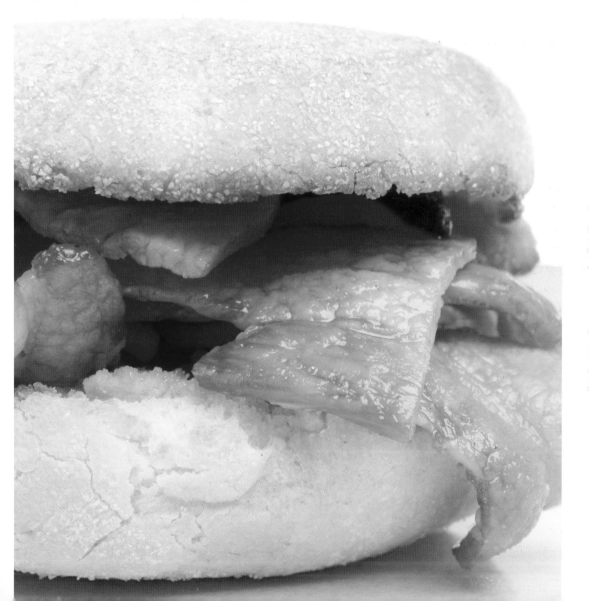

Counting Calories: Meat & Poultry

	Typical portion	Typical portion size	Calories per portion	Calories per 100 g/ml	Fat per 100 g/ml	Health rating (1–10)
Ham, gammon steak, grilled	1 medium	228 g/8 oz	453	**199**	9.9	5
Ham, honey roast	1 slice	20 g/¾ oz	25	**123**	3.8	4
Ham, honey roast, wafer thin	1 slice	10 g/¼ oz	11	**113**	3.2	5
Ham, lean	2 slices	36 g/1¼ oz	38	**104**	2.4	4
Ham, Parma	1 slice	12 g/⅜ oz	12	**109**	2.7	5
Ham, smoked, dry-cured	1 slice	28 g/1 oz	38	**137**	4.4	5
Ham, vegetarian	1 slice	10 g/¼ oz	25	**247**	14.7	3
Ham, wafer thin	1 slice	10 g/¼ oz	10	**101**	2.6	5
Pancetta	½ pack	65 g/2½ oz	212	**326**	28.7	4
Pork belly joint/slices, lean and fat, grilled	2 slices	120 g/4 oz	384	**320**	23.4	5
Pork diced, lean only, casseroled	¼ pack	140 g/5 oz	258	**184**	6.4	6
Pork fillet strips, lean, stir-fried	¼ pack	120 g/4 oz	218	**182**	5.9	6
Pork leg joint, lean and fat, raw	2 slices	140 g/5 oz	298	**213**	15.2	6
Pork leg joint, lean, medium-roasted	2 slices	140 g/5 oz	255	**182**	5.5	6
Pork leg joint, lean and fat, medium-roasted	2 slices	140 g/5 oz	301	**215**	10.2	6
Pork loin chops, raw, lean and fat	1	140 g/5 oz	378	**270**	21.7	5
Pork loin chops, barbecued, lean and fat	1	120 g/4 oz	306	**255**	15.8	5
Pork loin chops, lean, grilled	1	120 g/4 oz	220	**184**	6.4	6
Pork loin chops, lean and fat, grilled	1	120 g/4 oz	308	**257**	15.7	5
Pork loin chops, lean and fat, microwaved	1	140 g/5 oz	347	**248**	14.1	5
Pork loin chops, lean and fat, roasted	1	140 g/5 oz	421	**301**	19.3	5
Pork loin steaks, lean and fat, raw	1	140 g/5 oz	237	**169**	9.4	6

	Typical portion	Typical portion size	Calories per portion	Calories per 100 g/ml	Fat per 100 g/ml	Health rating (1–10)
Pork loin steaks, lean and fat, grilled	1	120 g/4 oz	237	**198**	7.6	6
Chicken						
Average meat, raw	2 slices	140 g/5 oz	151	**108**	2.1	6
Dark meat, raw	2 slices	140 g/5 oz	152	**109**	2.8	6
Light meat, raw	2 slices	140 g/5 oz	148	**106**	1.1	6
Average meat, roasted	2 slices	140 g/5 oz	249	**177**	7.5	6
Dark meat, roasted	2 slices	140 g/5 oz	274	**196**	10.9	6
Light meat, roasted	2 slices	140 g/5 oz	214	**153**	3.6	5
Breast, meat only, casseroled	1	140 g/5 oz	224	**160**	5.2	6
Breast, meat only, grilled	1	120 g/4 oz	178	**148**	2.2	6
Breast strips, stir-fried	¼ pack	140 g/5 oz	225	**161**	4.6	6
Breast, in breadcrumbs, fried	1	175 g/6 oz	392	**242**	12.7	3
Drumsticks, meat and skin, roasted	2	140 g/5 oz	259	**185**	9.1	5
Leg quarter, meat and skin, roasted	1	140 g/5 oz	330	**236**	16.9	5
Wing quarter, meat and skin, roasted	1	140 g/5 oz	316	**226**	14.1	4
Skin, dry, roasted/grilled	1 strip	60 g/2 oz	250	**501**	46.1	2
Turkey						
Average meat, raw	2 slices	140 g/5 oz	140	**105**	1.6	6
Light meat, raw	2 slices	140 g/5 oz	140	**105**	0.8	6
Dark meat, raw	2 slices	140 g/5 oz	146	**104**	2.5	6
Average meat, roasted	2 slices	140 g/5 oz	232	**166**	4.6	6
Light meat, roasted	2 slices	140 g/5 oz	214	**153**	2.0	6

	Typical portion	Typical portion size	Calories per portion	Calories per 100 g/ml	Fat per 100 g/ml	Health rating (1–10)
Dark meat, roasted	2 slices	140 g/5 oz	248	**177**	6.6	6
Breast, fillet, meat only, grilled	1	120 g/4 oz	186	**155**	1.7	6
Breast, fillet, strips, meat only, stir-fried	¼ pack	140 g/5 oz	230	**164**	4.5	5
Skin, dry, roasted	1 strip	60 g/2 oz	240	**481**	40.2	1
Duck						
Meat only, raw	2 slices	140 g/5 oz	192	**137**	6.5	6
Meat only, roasted	2 slices	140 g/5 oz	273	**195**	10.4	6
Meat, fat and skin, roasted	2 slices	140 g/5 oz	592	**423**	38.0	5
Crispy, Chinese-style	½ pack	120 g/4 oz	398	**331**	24.2	2
Other Meats, Fowl and Game						
Goose, meat, fat and skin, roasted	2 slices	140 g/5 oz	421	**301**	27.5	5
Grouse, meat only, roasted	2 breasts	140 g/5 oz	179	**128**	2.0	6
Guinea fowl, fresh, oven-ready	2 breasts	140 g/5 oz	188	**134**	6.2	5
Guinea fowl, boned and stuffed, oven-ready	2 breasts	120 g/4 oz	240	**200**	12.1	5
Partridge, meat only, roasted	2 breasts	140 g/5 oz	297	**212**	7.2	5
Pigeon, meat only, roasted	2 breasts	140 g/5 oz	262	**187**	7.9	6
Pheasant, meat only, roasted	2 breasts	120 g/4 oz	264	**220**	27.9	7
Hare, lean, raw	1 breast	120 g/4¼ oz	150	**125**	3.5	5
Hare, lean, stewed	1 breast	100 g/3½ oz	170	**170**	5.5	5
Rabbit, meat only, raw	½ pack	120 g/4 oz	165	**137**	5.5	5
Rabbit, meat only, stewed	½ pack	120 g/4 oz	137	**114**	3.2	5
Venison, roasted	2 slices	140 g/5 oz	231	**165**	2.5	7

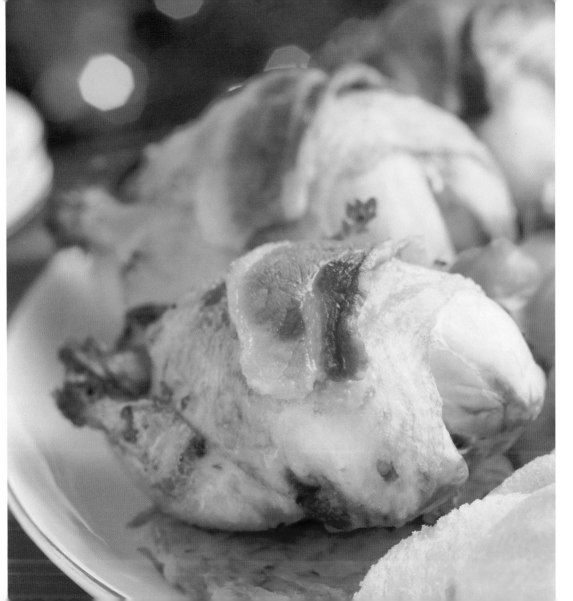

	Typical portion	Typical portion size	Calories per portion	Calories per 100 g/ml	Fat per 100 g/ml	Health rating (1–10)
Horse, raw	1 steak	140 g/5 oz	186	**133**	4.6	4
Kangaroo, raw	1 steak	150 g/5 oz	149	**98**	1.0	7
Kangaroo steak, grilled	1	150 g/5 oz	198	**132**	1.2	7
Offal						
Heart, lamb's, roasted	1	120 g/4 oz	271	**226**	13.9	4
Kidney, lamb's, fried	2	100 g/3½ oz	188	**188**	10.3	5
Kidney, ox, stewed	½ pack	100 g/3½ oz	138	**138**	4.4	5
Kidney, pig's, stewed	1	100 g/3½ oz	153	**153**	6.1	5
Liver, lamb's, fried	½ pack	100 g/3½ oz	237	**237**	12.9	4
Liver, calves', fried	½ pack	100 g/3½ oz	176	**176**	9.6	4
Liver, chicken, fried	¼ pack	50 g/2 oz	85	**169**	8.9	4
Liver, ox, stewed	½ pack	100 g/3½ oz	198	**198**	9.5	5
Liver, pig's, stewed	½ pack	100 g/3½ oz	189	**189**	8.1	5
Oxtail, stewed	½ pack	120 g/4 oz	291	**243**	13.4	4
Sweetbreads, raw	3 tbsp	80 g/3 oz	105	**131**	7.8	2
Sweetbreads, fried	3 tbsp	80 g/3 oz	174	**217**	11.4	2
Tongue, sheep's, stewed	¼ pack	90 g/3¼ oz	260	**289**	24.0	4
Tripe, dressed, raw	½ pack	100 g/3½ oz	33	**33**	0.5	3
Trotters and tails, boiled	n/a	n/a	n/a	**280**	22.3	2
Burgers – *see also* Takeaway & Convenience Food, page 244						
Beefburgers, chilled/frozen, raw	2	110 g/4 oz	320	**291**	24.7	4
Beefburgers, fried	2	110 g/4 oz	361	**329**	23.9	2

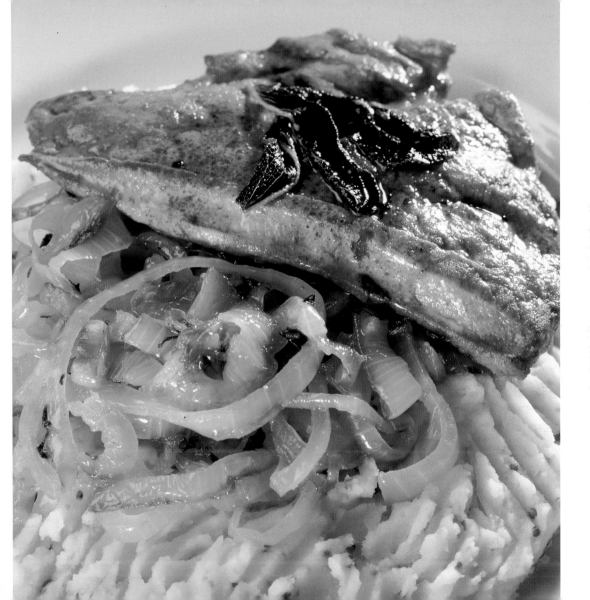

	Typical portion	Typical portion size	Calories per portion	Calories per 100 g/ml	Fat per 100 g/ml	Health rating (1–10)
Beefburgers, grilled	2	90 g/3¼ oz	294	**326**	24.4	4
Beefburgers, 100% meat	2	148 g/5 oz	462	**313**	22.4	5
Economy burgers, frozen, raw	2	100 g/3½ oz	261	**261**	21.2	3
Economy burgers, grilled	2	85 g/3 oz	232	**273**	19.3	3
Chicken burgers	1	46 g/1⅝ oz	115	**247**	15.1	4
Pork burger	1	122 g/4 oz	292	**239**	19.0	3
Turkey burger with crispy crumb	1	71 g/2½ oz	222	**313**	19.8	3
Venison burger	1	142 g/5 oz	170	**120**	4.9	5

Vegetable burgers – *see* Other Vegetable Products and Dishes, page 134

Meat Products

Bierwurst	1 slice	10 g/¼ oz	25	**252**	21.2	3
Biltong	1 slice	25 g/1 oz	64	**256**	4.0	3
Black pudding, dry-fried	2 slices	88 g/3⅛ oz	261	**297**	21.5	3
Chicken roll	2 slices	20 g/¾ oz	27	**131**	4.8	3
Chopped ham and pork, canned	2 slices	50 g/2 oz	98	**196**	24.2	3
Corned beef, canned	¼ pack	62 g/2⅛ oz	127	**205**	10.9	3
Frankfurter	2	160 g/5½ oz	459	**287**	25.4	2
Haggis, boiled	½	90 g/3¼ oz	279	**310**	21.7	3
Hash, barbecue beef	1 pack	200 g/7 oz	180	**90**	0.4	3
Hash, corned beef	1 pack	200 g/7 oz	240	**120**	6.3	3
Liver sausage	1 dssp	25 g/1 oz	56	**226**	16.7	2
Luncheon meat, canned	¼ can	28 g/1 oz	78	**279**	23.8	2

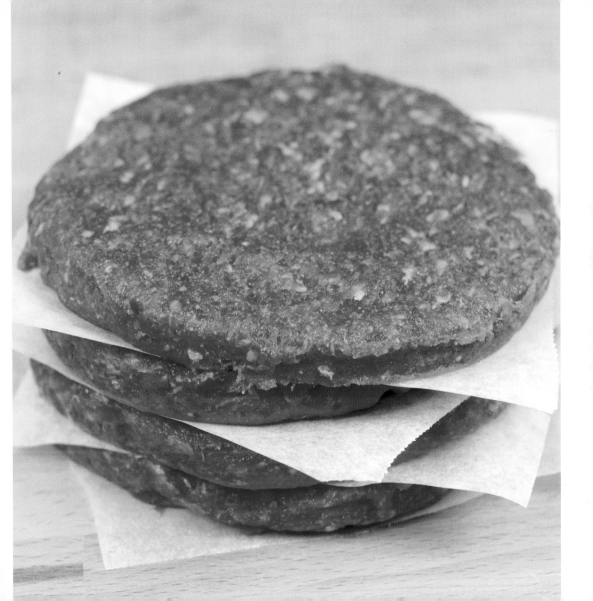

Counting Calories: Meat & Poultry

	Typical portion	Typical portion size	Calories per portion	Calories per 100 g/ml	Fat per 100 g/ml	Health rating (1–10)
Meat spread	1 dssp	25 g/1 oz	48	**192**	13.4	2
Meat samosas	1	75 g/3 oz	207	**272**	17.3	2
Paste, bacon and tomato	1 dssp	20 g/¾ oz	46	**232**	18.0	3
Paste, beef	1 dssp	20 g/¾ oz	39	**189**	13.2	3
Paste, chicken and ham	1 dssp	20 g/¾ oz	32	**158**	10.0	3
Pastrami	½ pack	40 g/1½ oz	51	**128**	3.6	4
Pastrami, turkey	½ pack	40 g/1½ oz	43	**107**	1.7	4
Pâté, Ardennes	1 tbsp	50 g/2 oz	143	**286**	24.0	3
Pâté, Ardennes, reduced fat	1 tbsp	50 g/2 oz	97	**194**	11.9	4
Pâté, Brussels mushroom	1 tbsp	50 g/2 oz	180	**360**	33.8	3
Pâté, Brussels, 50% less fat	1 tbsp	50 g/2 oz	112	**223**	16.0	4
Pâté, liver, chicken	1 tbsp	50 g/2 oz	117	**233**	18.4	3
Pâté, liver, pork	1 tbsp	50 g/2 oz	174	**348**	32.7	3
Pâté, meat, reduced fat	1 tbsp	50 g/2 oz	96	**191**	12.0	3
Potted beef	1 jar	75 g/3 oz	109	**145**	5.9	3
Polony	2 slices	28 g/1 oz	78	**281**	21.1	2
Salami, average	2 slices	28 g/1 oz	122	**438**	39.2	4
Salami, Danish	2 slices	28 g/1 oz	147	**524**	51.7	4
Salami, German	2 slices	28 g/1 oz	93	**333**	27.3	4
Salami, Milan	2 slices	28 g/1 oz	96	**342**	27.1	4
Salami, Spanish	2 slices	28 g/1 oz	96	**341**	23.5	4
Sausages, beef, chilled, grilled	2	124 g/4 oz	344	**278**	19.5	3

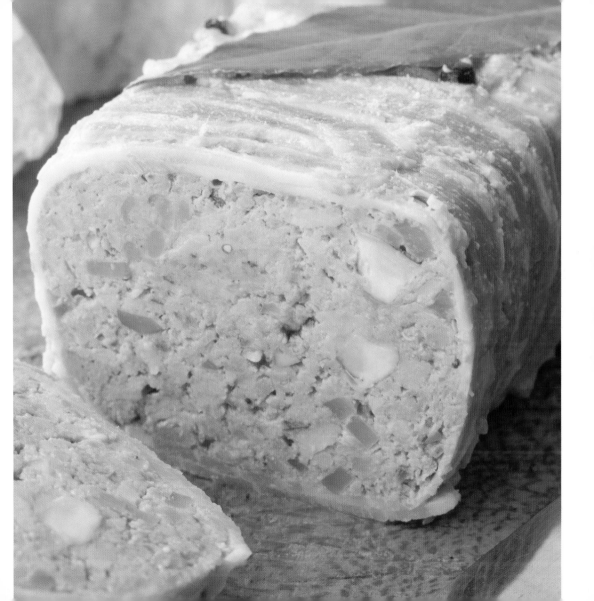

	Typical portion	Typical portion size	Calories per portion	Calories per 100 g/ml	Fat per 100 g/ml	Health rating (1–10)
Sausages, pork, raw	2	124 g/4 oz	383	**309**	25.0	3
Sausages, pork, chilled, fried	2	135 g/4¾ oz	415	**308**	23.9	2
Sausages, pork, chilled, grilled	2	135 g/4¾ oz	396	**294**	22.1	2
Sausages, reduced fat, chilled/frozen, grilled	2	102 g/3⅗ oz	235	**230**	13.8	3
Sausages, premium, chilled, grilled	2	102 g/3⅗ oz	297	**292**	22.4	3
Sausage and mash, meal for 1, chilled	1 pack	431 g/15⅕ oz	560	**130**	7.9	2
Sausage rolls, puff pastry	1	137 g/4⅚ oz	525	**383**	27.6	2
Scotch eggs	1	125 g/4 oz	301	**241**	16.0	3
Tongue slices	2 slices	28 g/1 oz	57	**201**	14.0	4
Turkey roll	2 slices	28 g/1 oz	47	**166**	9.0	3
Turkey ham roll	2 slices	28 g/1 oz	81	**108**	3.9	3
White pudding	2 slices	88 g/3⅑ oz	396	**450**	31.8	3
Meat Dishes and Meals – *see also* Takeaway and Convenience Food, from page 238						
Beef bourguignon	1 pack	225 g/8 oz	275	**122**	6.3	4
Beef bourguignon, made with lean beef	1 pack	225 g/8 oz	236	**105**	4.3	5
Beef en croute, ready to cook	1 pack	225 g/8 oz	506	**225**	13.0	3
Beef Wellington	1 pack	295/10⅓ oz	797	**270**	18.3	4
Casserole, beef, made with canned cook-in sauce	1 bowl	225 g/8 oz	306	**136**	6.5	5
Casserole, beef, with ale and dumplings	1 bowl	225 g/8 oz	356	**158**	7.3	4
Casserole, chicken, with dumplings, diet	½ pack	180 g/6⅓ oz	149	**83**	2.0	4
Casserole, pork, made with canned cook-in sauce	1 bowl	300 g/11 oz	463	**154**	7.8	3
Casserole, rabbit	1 pack	225/8 oz	230	**102**	5.1	5

	Typical portion	Typical portion size	Calories per portion	Calories per 100 g/ml	Fat per 100 g/ml	Health rating (1–10)
Casserole, sausage	1 pack	225/8 oz	371	**165**	10.9	4
Chasseur, beef and mashed potato	1 pack	450 g/1 lb	468	**104**	2.8	4
Chasseur, chicken	1 bowl	225 g/8 oz	219	**97**	4.1	3
Chicken in white sauce, canned	1 pack	300 g/11 oz	423	**141**	8.3	3
Chick. wings, marinated, chilled/frozen, barbecued	1 pack	225/8 oz	616	**274**	16.6	2
Chilli, beef	1 pack	225/8 oz	614	**273**	15.0	4
Chilli con carne, home-made	1 bowl	300 g/11 oz	363	**121**	7.5	4
Chilli con carne, chilled/frozen, reheated	1 pack	300 g/11 oz	465	**107**	2.7	4
Coq au vin	1 bowl	300 g/11 oz	465	**155**	11.0	3
Coronation chicken	1 tbsp	50 g/2 oz	182	**364**	31.7	2
Daube, beef and mashed potato	1 pack	402 g/14⅙ oz	346	**86**	2.0	4
Duck à l'orange, roasted	2 slices	140 g/5 oz	287	**205**	15.6	3
Duck and plum sauce, roasted	2 slices	140 g/5 oz	163	**116**	2.5	3
Duck in red wine sauce	2 slices	140 g/5 oz	211	**151**	7.7	3
Faggots in gravy, chilled/frozen, reheated	2 faggots	162 g/5½ oz	240	**148**	7.5	4
Gammon joint with orange glaze	2 slices	140 g/5 oz	200	**143**	7.0	4
Gammon steaks with cheese & mustard crust	1 steak	140 g/5 oz	182	**130**	4.3	4
Gammon steaks with cheese sauce	1 steak	140 g/5 oz	196	**140**	7.7	4
Gammon steaks with pineapple	1 steak	140 g/5 oz	182	**130**	1.4	4
Goulash, beef	1 bowl	300 g/11 oz	363	**121**	3.4	5
Goulash, healthy range	1 bowl	300 g/11 oz	219	**73**	1.7	5
Goulash, with tagliatelle	1 bowl	300 g/11 oz	345	**115**	2.3	4

Counting Calories: Meat & Poultry

	Typical portion	Typical portion size	Calories per portion	Calories per 100 g/ml	Fat per 100 g/ml	Health rating (1–10)
Hotpot, beef	1 bowl	300 g/11 oz	237	**79**	3.5	6
Hotpot, chicken	1 bowl	300 g/11 oz	255	**85**	2.7	6
Hotpot, lamb	1 bowl	300 g/11 oz	327	**109**	3.4	6
Hotpot, Lancashire	1 bowl	300 g/11 oz	294	**98**	3.9	6
Hotpot, sausage	1 bowl	300 g/11 oz	318	**106**	4.6	4
Jambalaya, American	½ pack	200 g/7 oz	314	**157**	7.0	4
Jambalaya, Cajun chicken	½ pack	200 g/7 oz	182	**91**	1.4	4
Jambalaya, spicy chicken	½ pack	200 g/7 oz	192	**96**	1.2	4
Kiev, chicken	1	100 g/3½ oz	247	**247**	16.5	3
Kiev, salmon	1	100 g/3½ oz	235	**235**	12.2	3
Kiev, turkey	1	100 g/3½ oz	221	**221**	11.8	3
Meatloaf, beef and pork	2 slices	100 g/3½ oz	275	**275**	22.0	5
Meatloaf, turkey and bacon	2 slices	100 g/3½ oz	178	**178**	9.9	5
Meatballs, beef	3 meatballs	108 g/3⅘ oz	278	**256**	19.8	5
Meatballs, canned in bolognese sauce	½ can	200 g/7 oz	33	**92**	2.9	4
Meatballs, canned in gravy	½ can	200 g/7 oz	29	**80**	2.6	4
Meatballs, canned in tomato sauce	½ can	200 g/7 oz	34	**94**	3.7	4
Meatballs, lamb	3 meatballs	108 g/3⅘ oz	295	**273**	21.0	5
Meatballs, pork	3 meatballs	108 g/3⅘ oz	155	**143**	5.3	5
Moussaka, lamb, healthy range	1 pack	350 g/12 oz	259	**74**	2.1	6
Moussaka, beef, healthy range	1 pack	350 g/12 oz	308	**88**	2.7	6
Moussaka, meat average, chilled/frozen	1 pack	350 g/12 oz	490	**140**	8.3	4

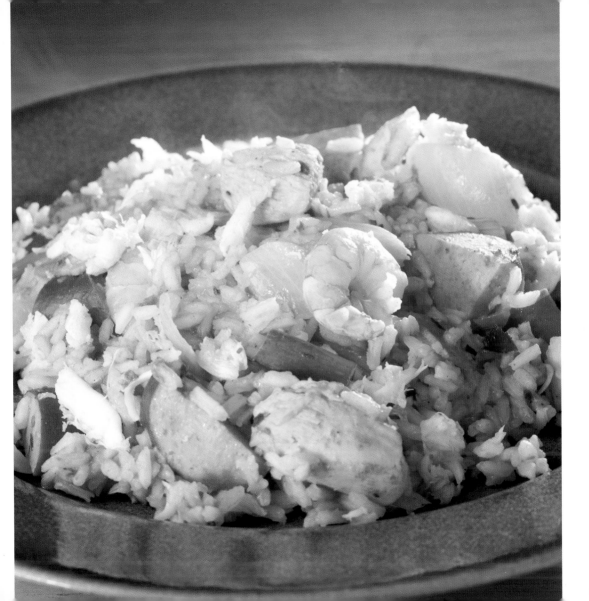

	Typical portion	Typical portion size	Calories per portion	Calories per 100 g/ml	Fat per 100 g/ml	Health rating (1–10)
Nachos, chilli beef	1 nacho	200 g/7 oz	208	**104**	5.0	4
Pies, meat – see Breads & Baked Products, page 198						
Pork belly, roasted with stuffing	3 slices	180 g/6⅓ oz	524	**291**	24.9	3
Roast dinner with beef	1 pack	283 g/10 oz	297	**105**	3.2	4
Shepherd's/cottage pie, chilled/frozen, reheated	1 pack	350 g/12 oz	389	**111**	5.4	4
Steak and chips	1 pack	450/1 lb	473	**105**	2.7	4
Steak, braised, and cabbage	1 pack	380 g/13⅓ oz	323	**85**	2.6	5
Steak, braised, and carrots	1 pack	200 g/7 oz	140	**70**	2.5	5
Steak, braised, and mashed potato	1 pack	450 g/1 lb	477	**106**	3.5	4
Stew, beef	1 bowl	225 g/8 oz	240	**107**	4.6	5
Stew, Irish	1 bowl	300 g/11 oz	354	**118**	6.2	4
Stew, Irish, canned	1 bowl	300 g/11 oz	273	**91**	5.1	3
Stew, Irish, made with lean lamb	1 bowl	300 g/11 oz	321	**107**	4.9	4
Stewed steak with onions and gravy, canned	1 can	410 g/14½ oz	537	**131**	7.0	4
Stifado, beef	1 pack	300/11 oz	411	**137**	5.8	5
Stroganoff, beef	1 bowl	200 g/7 oz	232	**116**	6.0	5
Stroganoff, chicken and mushroom	1 bowl	200 g/7 oz	200	**100**	2.0	5
Stroganoff, pork	1 bowl	200 g/7 oz	214	**107**	1.8	5
Toad-in-the-hole	½ pack	100 g/3½ oz	277	**277**	17.4	4
Turkey breast joint with sage and onion	2 slices	140 g/5 oz	141	**101**	1.7	5
Turkey breast with stuffing, cooked	2 slices	140 g/5 oz	146	**104**	2.0	4
Turkey with sausage meat stuffing	2 slices	140 g/5 oz	195	**139**	6.2	3

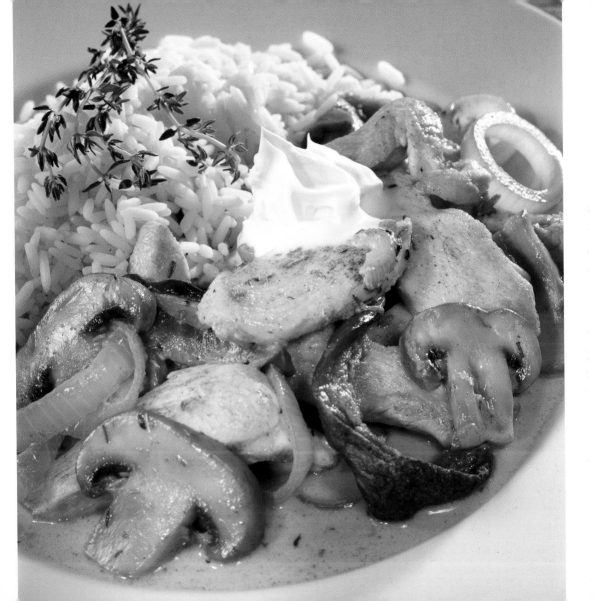

Fish & Seafood

	Typical portion	Typical portion size	Calories per portion	Calories per 100 g/ml	Fat per 100 g/ml	Health rating (1–10)
White Fish						
Bass, sea, raw	1 fillet	165 g/5½ oz	165	**100**	2.5	8
Bass, sea, farmed	1 fillet	140 g/5 oz	147	**105**	2.5	8
Cod, raw	1 fillet	165 g/5½ oz	132	**80**	0.7	8
Cod, baked	1 fillet	140 g/5 oz	135	**96**	1.2	8
Cod, poached	1 fillet	140 g/5 oz	131	**94**	1.1	8
Cod, grilled	1 fillet	125 g/4 oz	119	**95**	1.3	8
Cod in crumbs, fried in blended oil	1 fillet	150 g/5½ oz	352	**235**	14.3	5
Cod, dried, salted, boiled	1 fillet	50 g/2 oz	69	**138**	0.9	4
Coley, raw	1 fillet	165 g/5½ oz	135	**82**	1.0	8
Coley, steamed	1 fillet	140 g/5 oz	147	**105**	1.3	8
Crayfish, raw	6	165 g/5½ oz	110	**67**	0.8	7
Crayfish, tails, in brine	6	140 g/5 oz	72	**51**	0.7	5
Dab, raw	1 fillet	100 g/3½ oz	74	**74**	1.2	8
Dab, lightly dusted in flour and seasoning	1 fillet	112 g/4 oz	190	**170**	8.7	5
Dover sole, raw	1 fillet	160 g/5½ oz	143	**89**	1.8	8
Haddock, raw	1 fillet	165 g/5½ oz	134	**81**	0.6	8
Haddock in breadcrumbs	1 fillet	175 g/6 oz	355	**203**	9.9	4
Haddock, steamed	1 fillet	150 g/5 oz	147	**98**	0.6	8

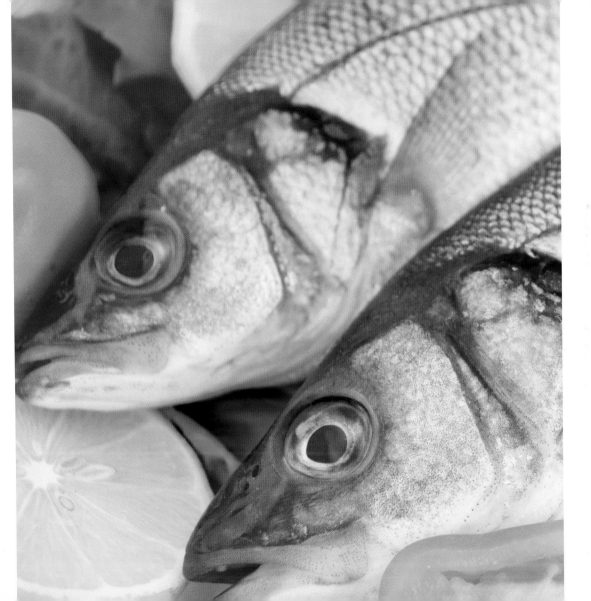

Counting Calories: Fish & Seafood

	Typical portion	Typical portion size	Calories per portion	Calories per 100 g/ml	Fat per 100 g/ml	Health rating (1–10)
Haddock, smoked, poached	1 fillet	150 g/5 oz	168	**112**	2.6	7
Hake in breadcrumbs	1 fillet	175 g/6 oz	355	**203**	9.9	4
Halibut, grilled	1 fillet	140 g/5 oz	170	**121**	2.2	8
Hoki, raw	1 steak	150 g/5 oz	128	**85**	1.9	7
Hoki, grilled	1 steak	150 g/5 oz	182	**121**	2.7	7
Lemon sole, raw	1 fillet	165 g/5½ oz	137	**83**	1.5	8
Lemon sole, steamed	1 fillet	140 g/5 oz	128	**91**	0.9	8
Monkfish, raw	1 steak	100 g/3½ oz	66	**66**	0.4	7
Monkfish, grilled	1 steak	100 g/3½ oz	96	**96**	0.6	7
Perch, raw	1 fillet	80 g/3 oz	75	**94**	1.6	7
Pollock, breaded	1 fillet	100 g/3½ oz	206	**206**	10.0	7
Mullet, grey, raw	1 fillet	140 g/5 oz	161	**115**	4.0	7
Mullet, grey, grilled	1 fillet	140 g/5 oz	210	**150**	5.2	7
Mullet, red, raw	1 fillet	140 g/5 oz	153	**109**	3.8	7
Mullet, red, grilled	1 fillet	100 g/3½ oz	121	**121**	4.4	7
Plaice, raw	1 fillet	165 g/5½ oz	130	**79**	1.4	8
Plaice, frozen, steamed	1 fillet	140 g/5 oz	129	**92**	1.5	8
Skate, raw	1 steak	100 g/3½ oz	64	**64**	0.4	7
Skate, grilled	1 steak	100 g/3½ oz	79	**79**	0.5	7
Turbot, raw	1 fillet	140 g/5 oz	133	**95**	2.7	8
Turbot, grilled	1 fillet	140 g/5 oz	170	**122**	3.5	8
Whiting, steamed	1 fillet	140 g/5 oz	129	**92**	0.9	8

	Typical portion	Typical portion size	Calories per portion	Calories per 100 g/ml	Fat per 100 g/ml	Health rating (1–10)
Oily Fish						
Anchovies, canned in olive oil	½ can drained	15 g/½ oz	30	**194**	11.3	5
Anchovy fillets, canned in olive oil	½ can	25 g/1 oz	57	**226**	14.0	5
Anchovies, salted	¼ small jar	25 g/1 oz	23	**93**	2.2	3
Catfish, cooked	1 fillet	75 g/3 oz	172	**229**	13.3	7
Eel, raw	1 fillet	75 g/3 oz	126	**168**	11.3	7
Eel, cooked or smoked, dry heat	1 fillet	75 g/3 oz	177	**236**	14.9	7
Eel, jellied	1 tub	100 g/3½ oz	98	**98**	7.1	5
Herring, raw	2	80 g/3 oz	152	**190**	13.2	8
Herring, grilled	2	75 g/3 oz	136	**181**	11.2	8
Kipper, raw	1 fillet	165 g/5½ oz	378	**229**	17.7	6
Kipper, grilled	1 fillet	140 g/5 oz	357	**255**	19.4	6
Mackerel, raw	1 fillet	165 g/5½ oz	363	**220**	16.1	8
Mackerel, grilled	1 fillet	140 g/5 oz	335	**239**	17.3	8
Mackerel, smoked	1 fillet	140 g/5 oz	496	**354**	30.9	6
Marlin, raw	1 steak	100 g/3½ oz	99	**99**	0.2	7
Marlin, chargrilled	1 steak	100 g/3½ oz	153	**153**	6.1	6
Marlin, smoked	1 steak	100 g/3½ oz	120	**120**	0.1	6
Pilchards, canned in tomato sauce	½ can	80 g/3 oz	116	**144**	8.1	5
Salmon, raw	1 fillet	140 g/5 oz	252	**180**	11.0	8
Salmon, grilled	1 fillet	125/4 oz	268	**215**	13.1	8
Salmon, steamed	1 fillet	140 g/5 oz	272	**194**	11.9	8

Counting Calories: Fish & Seafood

	Typical portion	Typical portion size	Calories per portion	Calories per 100 g/ml	Fat per 100 g/ml	Health rating (1–10)
Salmon, smoked	1 fillet	125 g/4 oz	178	**142**	4.5	7
Salmon, pink, canned in brine, flesh only, drained	½ can	110 g/4 oz	168	**153**	6.6	5
Sardines, canned in brine, drained	1 can	90 g/3¼ oz	155	**172**	9.6	5
Sardines, canned in oil, drained	1 can	90 g/3¼ oz	198	**220**	14.1	6
Sardines, canned in tomato sauce	1 can	90 g/3¼ oz	146	**162**	9.9	6
Sea bream, raw	1 fillet	100 g/3½ oz	96	**96**	2.9	8
Snapper, red, raw	1 fillet	100 g/3½ oz	90	**90**	1.3	7
Swordfish, grilled	1 fillet	125/4 oz	174	**139**	5.2	7
Tilapia, raw	1 fillet	100 g/3½ oz	95	**95**	1.0	7
Trout, brown, raw	1 fillet	140 g/5 oz	185	**132**	5.4	8
Trout, brown, steamed	1 fillet	120 g/4 oz	162	**135**	4.5	8
Trout, rainbow, raw	1 fillet	140 g/5 oz	178	**127**	5.1	8
Trout, rainbow, grilled	1 fillet	120 g/4 oz	162	**135**	5.4	8
Trout, rainbow, smoked	1 fillet	120 g/4 oz	168	**140**	5.6	7
Tuna steaks, raw	1 steak	140 g/5 oz	185	**132**	2.0	7
Tuna, bluefin, cooked, dry heat	1 steak	100 g/3 oz	184	**184**	6.3	7
Tuna, yellowfin, cooked, dry heat	1 steak	100 g/3 oz	139	**139**	1.2	7
Tuna, canned in brine, drained	½ can	75 g/3 oz	99	**99**	0.6	4
Tuna, canned in olive oil, drained	½ can	75 g/3 oz	190	**190**	9.6	6
Tuna, canned in sunflower oil, drained	½ can	75 g/3 oz	184	**184**	8.6	6

Seafood

	Typical portion	Typical portion size	Calories per portion	Calories per 100 g/ml	Fat per 100 g/ml	Health rating (1–10)
Clams, raw	20 small	180 g/6⅓ oz	133	**74**	1.0	5

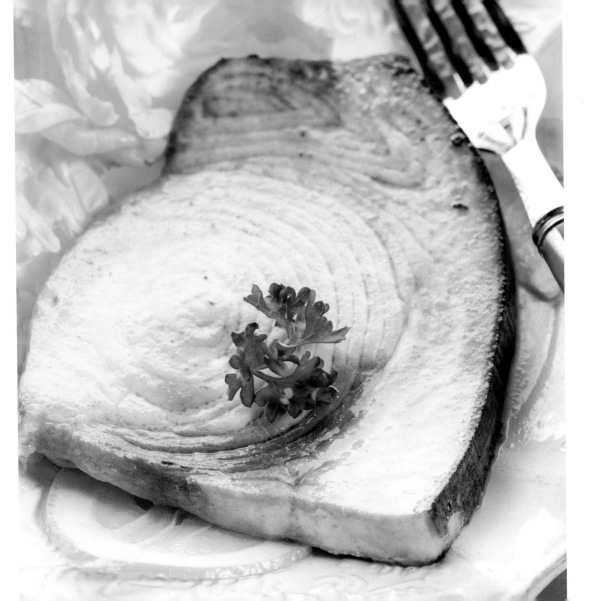

Counting Calories: Fish & Seafood

	Typical portion	Typical portion size	Calories per portion	Calories per 100 g/ml	Fat per 100 g/ml	Health rating (1–10)
Clams, in brine	20 small	180 g/6⅓ oz	142	**79**	0.6	5
Crab meat, raw	1 tbsp	40 g/1½ oz	40	**100**	0.6	7
Crab, boiled, meat only	1 tbsp	40 g/1½ oz	51	**128**	5.5	7
Crab, dressed	1 tbsp	40 g/1½ oz	62	**154**	7.9	7
Crab, canned in brine, drained	1 can	120 g/4 oz	92	**77**	0.5	4
Lobster, boiled	1 tbsp	40 g/1½ oz	41	**103**	1.6	7
Lobster, mini, breaded	1 pack	100 g/3½ oz	204	**204**	10.1	3
Lobster, dressed, canned	1 can	43 g/1½ oz	45	**105**	5.0	6
Lobster, dressed, chilled	1 pack	100 g/3½ oz	273	**273**	23.6	7
Octopus, raw	1 bowl	150 g/5 oz	124	**83**	1.3	5
Octopus chunks, in olive oil	1 can	111 g/4 oz	148	**133**	3.6	5
Prawns, boiled	10	30 g/1 oz	30	**99**	0.9	7
Prawns, cooked and peeled	3 tbsp	80 g/3 oz	62	**77**	0.6	7
Prawns, canned in brine	½ can	60 g/2 oz	58	**97**	1.0	4
King prawns, raw	1 bag	200 g/7 oz	145	**72**	0.9	7
Shrimps, canned in brine, drained	1 can	120 g/4 oz	113	**94**	1.2	4
Shrimps, boiled	1 tub	60 g/2 oz	70	**117**	2.4	6
Shrimps, dried	n/a	n/a	n/a	**245**	2.4	5
Shrimps, frozen	n/a	n/a	n/a	**73**	0.8	6
Cockles, boiled	10	40 g/1½ oz	21	**53**	0.6	5
Cockles, bottled in vinegar, drained	1 jar	90 g/3¼ oz	54	**60**	0.7	4
Mussels, raw	10	75 g/3 oz	66	**87**	2.5	6

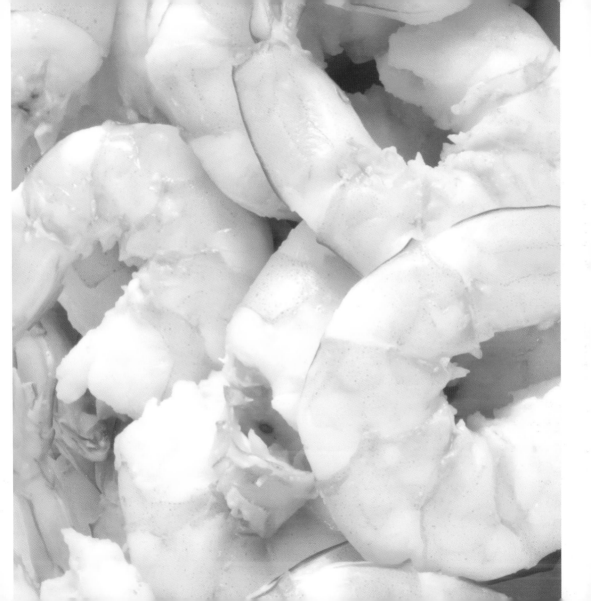

Counting Calories: Fish & Seafood

	Typical portion	Typical portion size	Calories per portion	Calories per 100 g/ml	Fat per 100 g/ml	Health rating (1–10)
Mussels, boiled	10	70 g/2½ oz	73	**104**	2.7	6
Mussels, pickled, drained	1 jar	90 g/3¼ oz	101	**112**	2.2	4
Oysters, raw	1 oyster	150 g/5 oz	98	**65**	1.3	6
Oysters, smoked, canned in sunflower oil, drained	1 can	85 g/3 oz	196	**230**	14.0	5
Squid, frozen, raw	1 bowl	150 g/5 oz	121	**81**	1.7	6
Squid pieces, in squid ink	1 can	120 g/4 oz	274	**228**	18.0	5
Whelks, boiled	1 tub	60 g/2 oz	54	**89**	1.2	5
Winkles, boiled	1 tub	60 g/2 oz	44	**72**	1.2	5

Fish Products

	Typical portion	Typical portion size	Calories per portion	Calories per 100 g/ml	Fat per 100 g/ml	Health rating (1–10)
Crabsticks	2	35 g/1¼ oz	24	**68**	0.4	4
Fishcakes, frozen	1 cake	85 g/3 oz	112	**132**	3.9	5
Fishcakes, fried in blended oil	1 cake	85 g/3 oz	185	**218**	13.4	3
Fishcakes, grilled	1 cake	85 g/3 oz	131	**154**	4.5	5
Fish fingers, frozen	1 finger	28 g/1 oz	48	**170**	7.8	4
Fish fingers, fried in blended oil	1 finger	28 g/1 oz	67	**238**	14.1	2
Fish fingers, grilled	1 finger	28 g/1 oz	56	**200**	8.9	4
Fish paste, crab	1 jar	30 g/1 oz	31	**104**	3.5	4
Fish paste, salmon	1 jar	30 g/1 oz	59	**195**	12.8	4
Fish paste, sardine and tomato	1 jar	30 g/1 oz	44	**146**	7.2	4
Hake goujons, baked	6	165 g/5½ oz	353	**214**	11.8	4
Lemon sole goujons, baked	6	165 g/5½ oz	308	**187**	14.6	4
Plaice goujons, baked	6	165 g/5½ oz	500	**304**	18.3	4

	Typical portion	Typical portion size	Calories per portion	Calories per 100 g/ml	Fat per 100 g/ml	Health rating (1–10)
Caviar	2 tsp	15 g/½ oz	14	**92**	4.7	5
Roe, cod, raw	2 tsp	15 g/½ oz	15	**96**	2.8	5
Roe, cod, hard, coated in batter, fried	½ can	100 g/3½ oz	189	**189**	11.8	2
Roe, cod, hard, fried in blended oil	½ can	100 g/3½ oz	202	**202**	11.9	2
Roe, herring, soft, raw	½ can	50 g/2 oz	46	**91**	2.6	5
Roe, herring, soft, fried in blended oil	½ can	50 g/2 oz	133	**265**	15.8	3
Taramasalata	¼ tub	50 g/2 oz	252	**504**	52.9	3
Taramasalata, reduced fat	¼ tub	50 g/2 oz	154	**307**	28.4	4
Pâté, smoked mackerel	1 tbsp	50 g/2 oz	189	**378**	35.3	4
Pâté, salmon	1 tbsp	50 g/2 oz	135	**272**	23.5	4
Pâté, smoked salmon	1 tbsp	50 g/2 oz	135	**270**	22.3	4
Pâté, tuna	1 tbsp	50 g/2 oz	118	**236**	18.6	3
Prawns, filo-wrapped and breaded	1 wrap	19 g/⅔ oz	45	**235**	13.0	3
Terrine, lobster and prawn	1 slice	80 g/3 oz	156	**195**	13.4	4
Terrine, poached salmon	1 slice	80 g/3 oz	247	**309**	27.1	4
Terrine, trout	1 slice	80 g/3 oz	184	**230**	17.9	4

Fish Meals – *see also* Takeaway & Convenience Food, page 238, 246, 248

	Typical portion	Typical portion size	Calories per portion	Calories per 100 g/ml	Fat per 100 g/ml	Health rating (1–10)
Cod in parsley sauce, frozen, boiled	1 fillet	175 g/6 oz	147	**84**	2.8	5
Fish steaks in butter sauce	1 steak	150 g/5 oz	115	**77**	2.8	4
Haddock en croute	1 piece	170 g/6 oz	432	**254**	16.9	4
Haddock Florentine	4 tbsp	200 g/7 oz	160	**80**	1.8	5
Haddock steak in butter sauce	1 steak	150 g/5 oz	133	**89**	3.7	4

Counting Calories: Fish & Seafood

	Typical portion	Typical portion size	Calories per portion	Calories per 100 g/ml	Fat per 100 g/ml	Health rating (1–10)
Haddock fillet in watercress sauce	1 fillet	150 g/5 oz	101	**67**	1.7	5
Haddock, smoked, with cheese crust	1 fillet	150 g/5 oz	222	**148**	9.5	4
Hake with tomato and chilli salsa	1 fillet	150 g/5 oz	90	**62**	0.9	5
Mornay cod	1 pack	150 g/5 oz	231	**154**	9.4	5
Mornay haddock	1 pack	150 g/5 oz	128	**85**	2.0	5
Mornay salmon, healthy range	1 pack	150 g/5 oz	135	**90**	1.7	6
Mussels in garlic butter sauce	1 pack	200 g/7 oz	158	**79**	5.1	4
Mussels in Thai sauce	1 pack	200 g/7 oz	108	**54**	2.5	5
Mussels in white wine sauce	1 pack	200 g/7 oz	176	**88**	3.7	3
Lobster thermador	½ pack	140 g/5 oz	287	**205**	13.7	4
Plaice with mushrooms and prawns	1 pack	170 g/6 oz	354	**208**	10.7	6
Plaice fillet with spinach and cheddar cheese	1 pack	154 g/5⅜ oz	222	**144**	8.6	5
Prawn cocktail	1 pot	80 g/3 oz	282	**353**	34.5	4
Prawn cocktail, reduced fat	1 pot	80 g/3 oz	104	**130**	7.5	5
Prawn creole with rice	½ pack	200 g/7 oz	136	**68**	1.1	5
Salmon en croute	½ pack	185 g/6½ oz	573	**310**	21.9	5
Salmon in lime and coriander	1 fillet	150 g/5 oz	189	**126**	2.9	6
Salmon in watercress sauce	1 fillet	150 g/5 oz	264	**176**	12.9	6
Salmon in white wine and parsley sauce	1 fillet	150 g/5 oz	246	**164**	11.3	4
Salmon with asparagus and rice	1 pack	400 g/14 oz	348	**87**	1.0	6
Seafood cocktail	2 tbsp	65 g/2½ oz	57	**87**	1.5	6
Sushi	1 pack	100 g/3½ oz	155	**155**	1.8	7

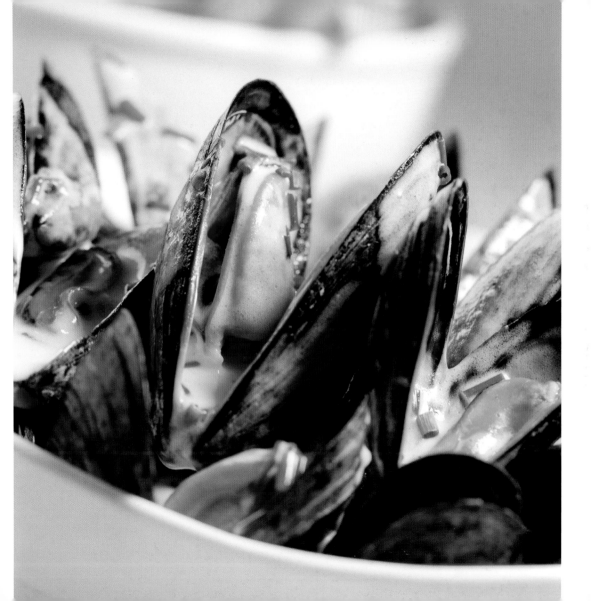

Vegetables

	Typical portion	Typical portion size	Calories per portion	Calories per 100 g/ml	Fat per 100 g/ml	Health rating (1–10)
Early Potatoes						
New potatoes, raw	5 small	145 g/5 oz	101	**70**	0.3	6
New potatoes, boiled in unsalted water	5 small	150 g/5 oz	113	**75**	0.3	6
New potatoes, in skins, boiled in unsalted water	5 small	150 g/5 oz	113	**75**	0.3	7
New potatoes, in skins, boiled in salted water	5 small	150 g/5 oz	99	**66**	0.3	5
New potatoes, canned, reheated, drained	5 small	150 g/5 oz	95	**63**	0.1	6
Main Crop Potatoes						
Old potatoes, raw	1 medium	175 g/6 oz	132	**75**	0.2	6
Old potatoes, flesh and skin, baked	1 medium	180 g/6⅓ oz	245	**136**	0.2	7
Old potatoes, flesh only, baked	1 medium	160 g/5½ oz	123	**77**	0.1	6
Old potatoes, boiled in unsalted water	5 small	150 g/5 oz	108	**72**	0.1	6
Old potatoes, boiled in salted water	5 small	150 g/5 oz	108	**72**	0.1	5
Old potatoes, mashed with butter	3 tbsp	100 g/3½ oz	104	**104**	4.3	5
Old potatoes, roasted in blended oil	5 small	150 g/5 oz	223	**149**	4.5	4
Old potatoes, roasted in corn oil	5 small	150 g/5 oz	223	**149**	4.5	3
Old potatoes, roasted in lard	5 small	150 g/5 oz	223	**149**	4.5	2
Beans – *see also* Nuts, Seeds & Pulses, page 74						
Broad beans, shelled, fresh	3 tbsp	80 g/3 oz	65	**81**	0.6	8
Broad beans, frozen, boiled in unsalted water	3 tbsp	80 g/3 oz	65	**81**	0.6	8

	Typical portion	Typical portion size	Calories per portion	Calories per 100 g/ml	Fat per 100 g/ml	Health rating (1–10)
Green/French beans, raw	3 tbsp	80 g/3 oz	20	**24**	0.5	8
Green/French beans, frozen, boiled in u/s water	3 tbsp	80 g/3 oz	20	**25**	0.1	8
Runner beans, raw	2 tbsp	80 g/3 oz	18	**22**	0.4	8
Runner beans, boiled in unsalted water	2 tbsp	80 g/3 oz	14	**18**	0.5	8
Runner beans and carrots, canned	2 tbsp	80 g/3 oz	20	**25**	0.1	8

Peas and Corn

	Typical portion	Typical portion size	Calories per portion	Calories per 100 g/ml	Fat per 100 g/ml	Health rating (1–10)
Alfalfa sprouts	½ bowl	80 g/3 oz	19	**24**	0.7	7
Mangetout peas, raw	3 tbsp	80 g/3 oz	26	**32**	0.2	8
Mangetout peas, boiled in salted water	3 tbsp	80 g/3 oz	21	**26**	0.1	6
Mangetout peas, stir-fried in blended oil	3 tbsp	80 g/3 oz	57	**71**	4.8	5
Marrowfat peas	3 tbsp	80 g/3 oz	70	**88**	0.6	5
Pea shoots	1 bowl	135 g/4¾ oz	12	**9**	0.3	8
Peas, raw	3 tbsp	80 g/3 oz	67	**83**	1.5	8
Peas, boiled in unsalted water	3 tbsp	80 g/3 oz	51	**79**	1.6	8
Peas, canned, reheated, drained	3 tbsp	80 g/3 oz	64	**80**	0.9	7
Peas, frozen, boiled in salted water	3 tbsp	80 g/3 oz	55	**69**	0.9	5
Peas, frozen, boiled in unsalted water	3 tbsp	80 g/3 oz	55	**69**	0.9	8
Peas, mushy, canned, reheated	3 tbsp	80 g/3 oz	65	**81**	0.7	4
Peas, processed, canned	3 tbsp	80 g/3 oz	64	**80**	0.8	6
Petit pois	3 tbsp	80 g/3 oz	42	**53**	0.7	8
Petit pois, frozen, boiled in unsalted water	3 tbsp	80 g/3 oz	39	**49**	0.9	8
Processed peas, canned, reheated, drained	3 tbsp	80 g/3 oz	79	**99**	0.7	6

Counting Calories: Vegetables

	Typical portion	Typical portion size	Calories per portion	Calories per 100 g/ml	Fat per 100 g/ml	Health rating (1–10)
Sugar snap peas	3 tbsp	80 g/3 oz	27	**34**	0.2	8
Sweetcorn on the cob, whole, boiled in u/s water	1 cob	100 g/3½ oz	111	**111**	2.3	8
Sweetcorn, baby, canned, drained	½ can	125 g/4 oz	29	**23**	0.4	8
Sweetcorn, kernels, canned, reheated, drained	½ can	125 g/4 oz	153	**122**	1.2	8

Root Vegetables

Beetroot, raw	1 medium	50 g/2 oz	18	**36**	0.1	8
Beetroot, boiled in salted water	3 tbsp	80 g/3 oz	37	**46**	0.1	5
Beetroot, pickled, drained	3 tbsp	80 g/3 oz	35	**43**	0.2	4
Breadfruit, raw	¼	80 g/3 oz	76	**95**	0.3	7
Breadfruit, canned and drained	½ can	75 g/3 oz	50	**66**	0.2	7
Carrots, old, raw	2 medium	50 g/2 oz	17	**35**	0.3	9
Carrots, old, boiled in unsalted water	2	80 g/3 oz	19	**24**	0.4	9
Carrots, young, raw	5	80 g/3 oz	24	**30**	0.5	9
Carrots, young, boiled in unsalted water	5	80 g/3 oz	18	**22**	0.4	9
Carrots, young, canned, reheated, drained	5	80 g/3 oz	16	**20**	0.3	9
Cassava, raw	1 slice	50 g/2 oz	81	**142**	0.2	7
Cassava, baked	3 tbsp	80 g/3 oz	124	**155**	0.2	7
Cassava, boiled in unsalted water	3 tbsp	80 g/3 oz	104	**130**	0.2	7
Cassava, steamed	3 tbsp	80 g/3 oz	115	**142**	0.2	7
Celeriac, raw	3 tbsp	80 g/3 oz	34	**42**	0.3	7
Celeriac, boiled in salted water	3 tbsp	80 g/3 oz	12	**15**	0.5	7
Fennel, Florence, raw	1 slice	28 g/1 oz	4	**12**	0.2	7

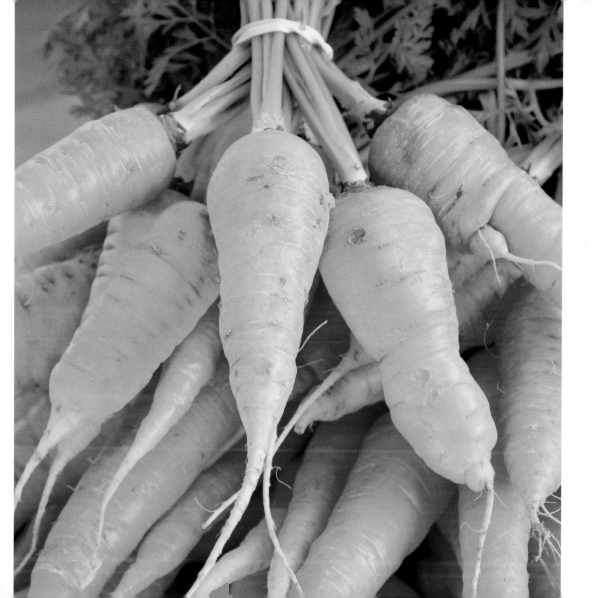

Counting Calories: Vegetables

	Typical portion	Typical portion size	Calories per portion	Calories per 100 g/ml	Fat per 100 g/ml	Health rating (1–10)
Fennel, Florence, boiled in salted water	1 slice	28 g/1 oz	9	**11**	0.2	7
Parsnip, raw	1 medium	50 g/2 oz	32	**64**	1.1	8
Parsnip, boiled in salted water	3 tbsp	80 g/3 oz	53	**66**	1.2	5
Parsnip, boiled in unsalted water	3 tbsp	80 g/3 oz	53	**66**	1.2	8
Parsnip, roasted	3 tbsp	80 g/3 oz	96	**120**	6.4	5
Parsnip, honey roasted	3 tbsp	80 g/3 oz	152	**190**	7.5	3
Parsnip, roasting, retail	3 tbsp	80 g/3 oz	82	**103**	4.2	3
Radish, red, raw	3 tbsp	80 g/3 oz	10	**12**	0.2	7
Swede, raw	3 tbsp	80 g/3 oz	17	**21**	0.3	8
Swede, boiled	3 tbsp	80 g/3 oz	9	**11**	0.1	8
Swede, mashed	3 tbsp	80 g/3 oz	44	**55**	1.2	7
Sweet potato, raw	½	50 g/2 oz	44	**87**	0.3	8
Sweet potato, boiled in unsalted water	3 tbsp	80 g/3 oz	67	**84**	0.3	8
Sweet potato, steamed	3 tbsp	80 g/3 oz	67	**84**	0.3	8
Turnip, raw	¼	80 g/3 oz	18	**23**	0.3	7
Turnip, boiled in unsalted water	3 tbsp	80 g/3 oz	10	**12**	0.2	7
Yam, raw	1	80 g/3 oz	91	**114**	0.3	8
Yam, boiled in unsalted water	3 tbsp	80 g/3 oz	107	**133**	0.3	8

Cabbage Family

	Typical portion	Typical portion size	Calories per portion	Calories per 100 g/ml	Fat per 100 g/ml	Health rating (1–10)
Broccoli, green, raw	2 florets	80 g/3 oz	27	**33**	0.9	8
Broccoli, green, boiled in unsalted water	2 florets	80 g/3 oz	19	**24**	0.8	8
Brussels sprouts, raw	8	80 g/3 oz	34	**42**	1.4	8

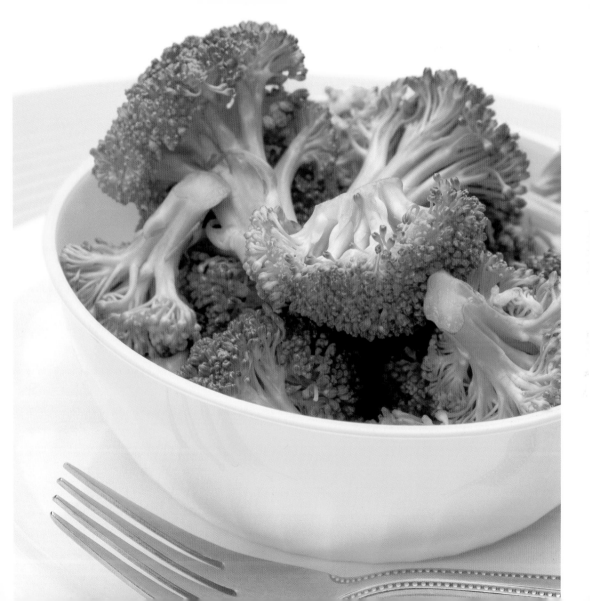

Counting Calories: Vegetables

	Typical portion	Typical portion size	Calories per portion	Calories per 100 g/ml	Fat per 100 g/ml	Health rating (1–10)
Brussels sprouts, boiled in unsalted water	8	80 g/3 oz	28	**35**	1.3	8
Brussels sprouts, frozen, boiled in u/s water	8	80 g/3 oz	28	**35**	1.3	8
Cabbage, average, raw	¼	50 g/2 oz	13	**26**	0.4	8
Cabbage, avergae, boiled in unsalted water	3 tbsp	80 g/3 oz	13	**16**	0.4	8
Cabbage, white, raw	⅙	80 g/3 oz	22	**27**	0.2	8
Cauliflower, raw	2 florets	80 g/3 oz	27	**34**	0.9	7
Cauliflower, boiled in unsalted water	2 florets	80 g/3 oz	22	**28**	0.9	7
Curly kale, raw	3 tbsp	80 g/3 oz	26	**33**	1.6	8
Curly kale, boiled in salted water	3 tbsp	80 g/3 oz	19	**24**	1.1	8
Kohlrabi, raw	⅓	50 g/2 oz	12	**23**	0.2	7
Kohlrabi, boiled in salted water	3 tbsp	80 g/3 oz	14	**18**	0.2	7
Spring greens, raw	3 tbsp	80 g/3 oz	26	**33**	1.0	8
Spring greens, boiled in unsalted water	3 tbsp	80 g/3 oz	16	**20**	0.7	8

Leaf Vegetables

Chard, Swiss, raw	3 tbsp	80 g/3 oz	15	**19**	0.2	7
Chard, Swiss, boiled in unsalted water	3 tbsp	80 g/3 oz	16	**20**	0.1	7
Chicory, raw	n/a	n/a	n/a	**11**	0.6	6
Endive, raw	1 slice	28 g/1 oz	4	**13**	0.2	7
Lettuce, average, raw	1 bowl	150 g/5 oz	21	**14**	0.5	6
Lettuce, iceberg, raw	1 bowl	150 g/5 oz	20	**13**	0.3	6
Lettuce/salad mix, retail, bagged	1 bowl	150 g/5 oz	33	**22**	0.3	6
Mustard cress, raw	1 handful	28 g/1 oz	4	**13**	0.6	7

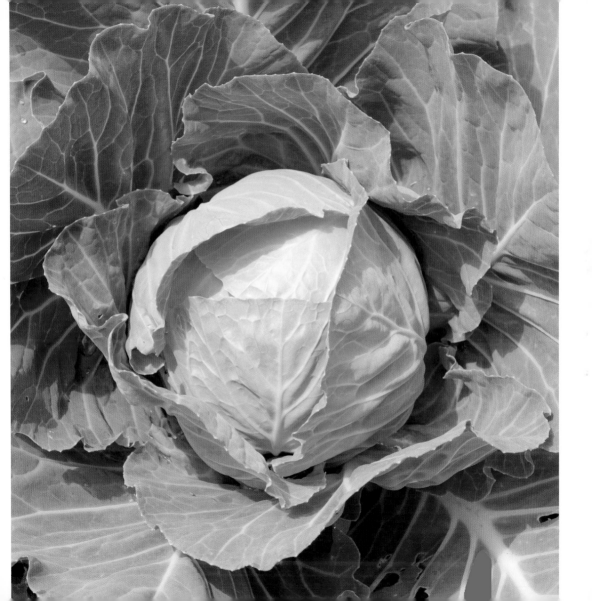

Counting Calories: Vegetables

	Typical portion	Typical portion size	Calories per portion	Calories per 100 g/ml	Fat per 100 g/ml	Health rating (1–10)
Pak choi, raw	½	60 g/2 oz	60	**13**	0.2	7
Rocket, fresh, raw	1 handful	28 g/1 oz	7	**25**	0.7	6
Seaweed, crispy	2 tbsp	30 g/1 oz	195	**651**	61.9	4
Seaweed, Irish moss, raw	1 handful	50 g/2 oz	4	**8**	0.2	6
Seaweed, Kombu, dried, raw	1 tbsp	10 g/¼ oz	4	**43**	1.6	6
Seaweed, Nori, dried, raw	1 tbsp	10 g/¼ oz	14	**136**	1.5	6
Seaweed, Wakame, dried, raw	1 tbsp	10 g/¼ oz	7	**71**	2.4	6
Spinach, raw	3 tbsp	80 g/3 oz	20	**25**	0.8	8
Spinach, boiled in unsalted water	3 tbsp	80 g/3 oz	15	**19**	0.8	8
Spinach, frozen, boiled in unsalted water	3 tbsp	80 g/3 oz	17	**21**	0.8	8
Watercress, raw	1 handful	28 g/1 oz	7	**22**	1.0	8

Squashes and Cucumber

	Typical portion	Typical portion size	Calories per portion	Calories per 100 g/ml	Fat per 100 g/ml	Health rating (1–10)
Courgette, raw	1 medium	50 g/2 oz	9	**18**	0.4	7
Courgette, boiled in unsalted water	3 tbsp	80 g/3 oz	15	**19**	0.4	7
Courgette, fried in corn oil	3 tbsp	80 g/3 oz	50	**63**	4.8	3
Cucumber, raw	¼	50 g/2 oz	5	**10**	0.1	6
Gherkins, pickled, drained	1	40 g/1 oz	5.6	**14**	0.1	3
Gourd, Kerala, raw	1	50 g/2 oz	6	**11**	0.2	7
Marrow, raw	⅛	80 g/3 oz	9	**12**	0.2	7
Marrow, boiled in unsalted water	3 tbsp	80 g/3 oz	7	**9**	0.2	7
Pumpkin, raw	3 tbsp	80 g/3 oz	10	**13**	0.2	8
Pumpkin, boiled in salted water	3 tbsp	80 g/3 oz	10	**13**	0.3	5

	Typical portion	Typical portion size	Calories per portion	Calories per 100 g/ml	Fat per 100 g/ml	Health rating (1–10)
Squash, butternut, raw	¼	80 g/3 oz	30	**37**	0.1	9
Squash, butternut, baked	3 tbsp	80 g/3 oz	26	**32**	0.1	9
Squash, acorn, raw	¼	80 g/3 oz	32	**40**	0.1	9
Squash, acorn, baked	3 tbsp	80 g/3 oz	45	**56**	0.1	9
Squash, spaghetti	3 tbsp	80 g/3 oz	30	**37**	0.1	8
Onion Family						
Garlic, raw	1 clove	3 g/⅒ oz	3	**98**	0.6	7
Leeks, raw	1 large	80 g/3 oz	17	**22**	0.5	8
Leeks, boiled in unsalted water	3 tbsp	80 g/3 oz	17	**21**	0.7	8
Onions, raw	3 tbsp	80 g/3 oz	25	**31**	0.2	8
Onions, raw, dried	1 tbsp	32 g/1⅛ oz	100	**313**	1.7	7
Onions, baked	3 tbsp	80 g/3 oz	82	**103**	0.6	8
Onions, boiled in salted water	3 tbsp	80 g/3 oz	14	**17**	0.1	7
Onions, fried in corn oil	3 tbsp	80 g/3 oz	131	**164**	11.2	3
Onions, pickled, average, drained	1	15 g/½ oz	4	**24**	0.2	4
Onions, pickled, cocktail/silverskin, drained	5	15 g/½ oz	3	**15**	0.1	4
Onions, spring, bulbs and tops, raw	3 tbsp	80 g/3 oz	18	**23**	0.5	8
Shallots, raw	3 tbsp	80 g/3 oz	16	**20**	0.2	8
Shallots, pickled	1 bulb	18 g/⅝ oz	8	**77**	0.1	5
Soft Vegetables						
Aubergine, raw	½	80 g/3 oz	12	**15**	0.4	7
Aubergine, fried in corn oil	3 tbsp	80 g/3 oz	242	**302**	31.9	4

Counting Calories: Vegetables

	Typical portion	Typical portion size	Calories per portion	Calories per 100 g/ml	Fat per 100 g/ml	Health rating (1–10)
Aubergine, fried in butter	3 tbsp	80 g/3 oz	242	**302**	31.9	4
Peppers, chilli, bird's-eye	3 tbsp	80 g/3 oz	16	**20**	0.6	9
Peppers, chilli, green, raw	3 tbsp	80 g/3 oz	16	**20**	0.6	8
Peppers, capsicum, green, raw	3 tbsp	80 g/3 oz	12	**15**	0.3	7
Peppers, green, boiled in salted water	3 tbsp	80 g/3 oz	14	**18**	0.5	7
Peppers, capsicum, red, raw	3 tbsp	80 g/3 oz	26	**32**	0.4	9
Peppers, capsicum, red, boiled in salted water	3 tbsp	80 g/3 oz	27	**34**	0.4	8
Tomatoes, raw	1 medium	100 g/3½ oz	17	**17**	0.3	8
Tomatoes, fried in corn oil	1 medium	100 g/3½ oz	91	**91**	7.7	3
Tomatoes, grilled	1 medium	100 g/3½ oz	20	**20**	0.3	7
Tomatoes, canned, whole contents	½ can	200 g/7 oz	32	**16**	0.1	7
Tamarillos, fresh, raw	1 fruit	50 g/2 oz	14	**28**	0.3	7
Other Vegetables						
Artichoke, raw, fresh	3 tbsp	80 g/3 oz	38	**47**	0.2	6
Artichoke, hearts, drained	3 tbsp	80 g/3 oz	23	**29**	0.1	6
Artichoke, hearts, marinated and grilled	3 tbsp	80 g/3 oz	91	**114**	10.0	4
Asparagus, raw	5 spears	125 g/4 oz	32	**25**	0.6	8
Asparagus, boiled in salted water	5 spears	125 g/4 oz	32	**26**	0.8	5
Asparagus, canned, reheated and drained	½ can	125 g/4 oz	31	**24**	0.5	7
Bamboo shoots, canned	½ can	60 g/2/ oz	5	**9**	0.1	5
Caperberries	1 tsp	7 g/¼ oz	2	**17**	0.5	5
Celery, raw	1 stick	10 g/¼ oz	1	**7**	0.2	5

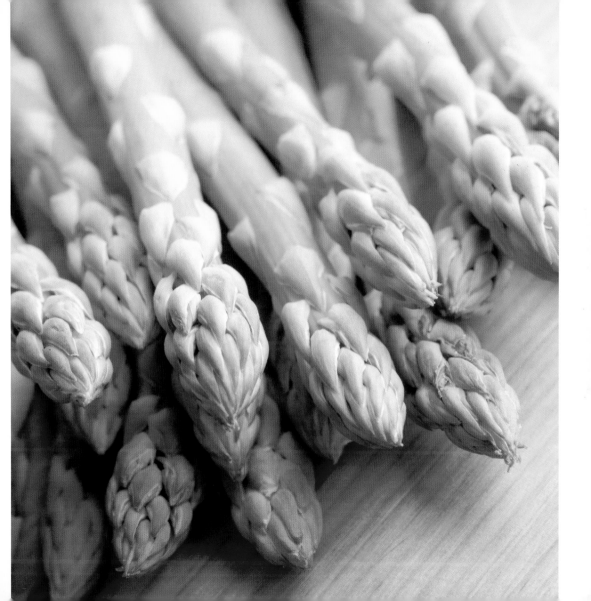

	Typical portion	Typical portion size	Calories per portion	Calories per 100 g/ml	Fat per 100 g/ml	Health rating (1–10)
Celery, boiled in salted water	3 tbsp	80 g/3 oz	6	**8**	0.3	4
Lemongrass stalks	1 stalk	13 g/½ oz	12	**99**	0.5	6
Mixed vegetables, frozen, boiled in salted water	3 tbsp	80 g/3 oz	34	**42**	0.5	7
Mushrooms, common, raw	3 tbsp	80 g/3 oz	10	**13**	0.5	6
Mushrooms, common, fried in butter	3 tbsp	80 g/3 oz	126	**157**	16.2	4
Mushrooms, common, fried in corn oil	3 tbsp	80 g/3 oz	126	**157**	16.2	3
Okra, raw	4	50 g/2 oz	16	**31**	1.0	5
Okra, boiled in unsalted water	3 tbsp	80 g/3 oz	22	**28**	0.9	5
Okra, fried in corn oil	3 tbsp	80 g/3 oz	215	**269**	26.1	3
Plantain, boiled in unsalted water	3 tbsp	80 g/3 oz	90	**112**	0.2	7
Plantain, ripe, fried in vegetable oil	3 tbsp	80 g/3 oz	214	**267**	9.2	3
Quorn, pieces	3 tbsp	80 g/3 oz	74	**92**	3.2	4

Potato Products – *see also* Other Vegetable Products and Dishes, page 138

	Typical portion	Typical portion size	Calories per portion	Calories per 100 g/ml	Fat per 100 g/ml	Health rating (1–10)
Chips, home-made, fried in blended oil	3 tbsp	80 g/3 oz	151	**189**	6.7	2
Chips, home-made, fried in corn oil	3 tbsp	80 g/3 oz	151	**189**	6.7	1
Chips, home-made, fried in dripping	3 tbsp	80 g/3 oz	151	**189**	6.7	1
Chips, retail, fried in blended oil	3 tbsp	80 g/3 oz	191	**2**	12.4	1
Chips, retail, fried in dripping	3 tbsp	80 g/3 oz	191	**239**	12.4	1
Chips, retail, fried in vegetable oil	3 tbsp	80 g/3 oz	191	**239**	12.4	1
Chips, fine cut, frozen, fried in blended oil	3 tbsp	80 g/3 oz	291	**364**	21.3	1
Chips, fine cut, frozen, fried in corn oil	3 tbsp	80 g/3 oz	291	**364**	21.3	1
Chips, straight cut, frozen, fried in blended oil	3 tbsp	80 g/3 oz	218	**273**	13.5	1

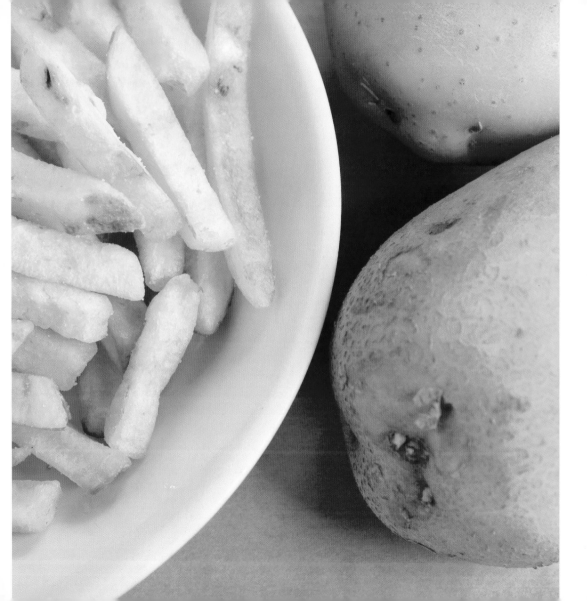

Counting Calories: Vegetables

	Typical portion	Typical portion size	Calories per portion	Calories per 100 g/ml	Fat per 100 g/ml	Health rating (1–10)
Chips, straight cut, frozen, fried in corn oil	3 tbsp	80 g/3 oz	218	**273**	13.5	1
Chips, straight cut, frozen, fried in dripping	3 tbsp	80 g/3 oz	291	**364**	21.3	1
Chips, oven, 5% fat, frozen	3 tbsp	80 g/3 oz	133	**166**	4.2	5
Chips, oven, frozen, baked	3 tbsp	80 g/3 oz	130	**162**	4.2	5
Chips, oven, crinkle cut, 5% fat, frozen	3 tbsp	80 g/3 oz	108	**134**	3.6	5
Chips, oven, crinkle cut, 5% fat, baked	3 tbsp	80 g/3 oz	131	**163**	4.3	5
Chips, microwave, cooked	3 tbsp	80 g/3 oz	177	**221**	9.6	3
French fries, retail	3 tbsp	80 g/3 oz	224	**280**	15.5	1
Hash browns, frozen, oven baked	1 piece	38 g/1½ oz	80	**214**	11.4	4
Potato powder, instant, made up with water	3 tbsp	80 g/3 oz	46	**57**	0.1	2
Potato powder, instant, made up with whole milk	3 tbsp	80 g/3 oz	61	**76**	1.2	4
Potato croquettes	1	41 g/1½ oz	68	**165**	8.8	4
Potato croquettes, fried in blended oil	1	80 g/3 oz	171	**214**	13.1	2
Potato and parsnip croquettes	1	41 g/1½ oz	86	**210**	9.9	5
Potato fritters, battered, cooked	3 tbsp	80 g/3 oz	148	**185**	8.5	1
Rosti, oven baked	1 rosti	100 g/3½ oz	194	**194**	9.3	6
Potato waffles, grilled	1 waffle	60 g/2 oz	110	**183**	10.1	3
Potato cakes	1 cake	70 g/2½ oz	127	**180**	1.7	3
Potatoes, fried, crispy	3 tbsp	80 g/3 oz	132	**165**	7.1	2
Potato fritters, oven baked	1	20 g/¾ oz	29	**145**	8.0	2
Potato fritters with sweetcorn	1	30 g/1 oz	68	**225**	12.6	2

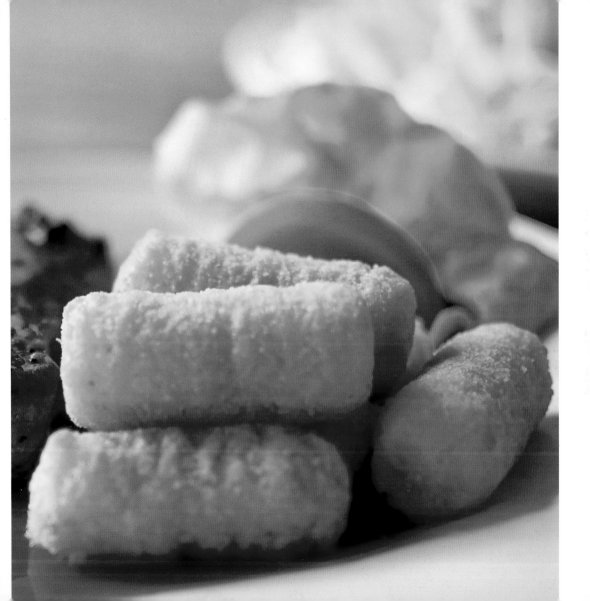

	Typical portion	Typical portion size	Calories per portion	Calories per 100 g/ml	Fat per 100 g/ml	Health rating (1–10)
Other Vegetable Products and Dishes						
Bake, aubergine and mozzarella, healthy range	½ pack	200 g/7 oz	144	**72**	3.4	6
Bake, Mediterranean vegetable	½ pack	200 g/7 oz	380	**190**	10.0	5
Bake, roast onion and potato, healthy range	½ pack	200 g/7 oz	144	**75**	1.3	5
Bake, vegetable	1 pack	225 g/8 oz	295	**131**	7.2	5
Bubble and squeak	3 tbsp	80 g/3 oz	64	**80**	3.3	5
Bubble and squeak, fried in vegetable oil	3 tbsp	80 g/3 oz	100	**125**	9.1	3
Burger, bean, Mexican style	1	114 g/4 oz	250	**220**	10.6	4
Burger, bean, soya, fried in vegetable oil	1	56 g/2 oz	109	**193**	11.0	3
Burger, black bean	1	88 g/3⅛ oz	169	**193**	11.5	4
Burger, mushroom	1	88 g/3⅛ oz	125	**143**	6.3	4
Burger, spicy bean, healthy range	1	85 g/3 oz	123	**145**	23.3	4
Burger, spicy vegetable	1	56 g/2 oz	108	**193**	11.0	4
Burger, vegetable	1	114 g/4 oz	240	**211**	10.2	4
Burger, vegetable with tofu	1	56 g/2 oz	104	**186**	8.3	4
Casserole, bean and lentil	1 bowl	300 g/11 oz	210	**70**	0.4	6
Casserole, vegetable	1 bowl	300 g/11 oz	156	**52**	0.4	6
Casserole, vegetable and lentil	1 bowl	300 g/11 oz	204	**68**	2.0	6
Cauliflower cheese made with semi-skimmed milk	3 tbsp	80 g/3 oz	80	**100**	6.4	5
Cauliflower cheese made with skimmed milk	3 tbsp	80 g/3 oz	78	**97**	6.0	5
Cauliflower cheese made with whole milk	3 tbsp	80 g/3 oz	84	**105**	6.9	5
Chilli, vegetable	1 pack	225 g/8 oz	126	**56**	0.6	6

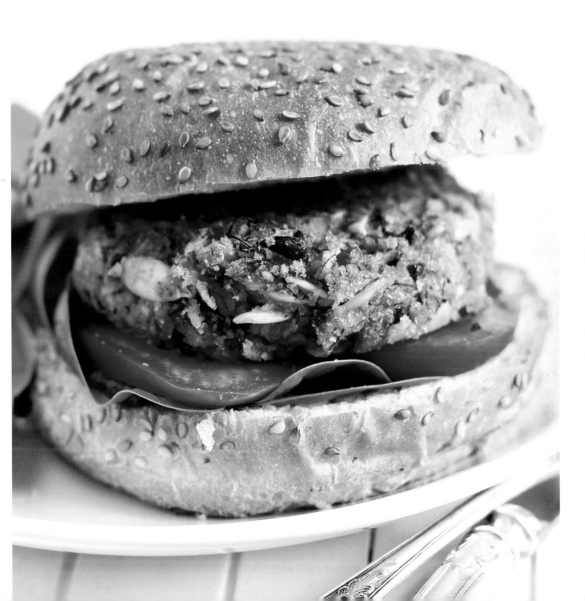

Counting Calories: Vegetables

	Typical portion	Typical portion size	Calories per portion	Calories per 100 g/ml	Fat per 100 g/ml	Health rating (1–10)
Coleslaw	2 tbsp	80 g/3 oz	48	**60**	2.7	4
Coleslaw, apple	2 tbsp	80 g/3 oz	152	**190**	16.6	5
Coleslaw, cheese	2 tbsp	80 g/3 oz	260	**325**	33.5	4
Coleslaw, deli style	2 tbsp	80 g/3 oz	84	**105**	9.7	4
Coleslaw, reduced fat	2 tbsp	80 g/3 oz	164	**205**	20.0	5
Coleslaw, with mayonnaise	2 tbsp	50 g/2 oz	129	**258**	26.4	4
Coleslaw, with reduced calorie dressing	2 tbsp	50 g/2 oz	34	**67**	4.5	4
Courgette and tomato bake	½ pack	200 g/7 oz	416	**208**	13.0	6
Crudités selection	1 pack	250 g/9 oz	75	**30**	0.4	6
Cutlets, nut, fried in blended oil	1	88 g/3⅛ oz	254	**289**	22.3	3
Cutlets, nut, grilled	1	88 g/3⅛ oz	187	**212**	13.0	5
Flan, vegetable	¼	90 g/3¼ oz	203	**226**	14.5	3
Garlic butter	1 knob	28 g/1 oz	192	**686**	75.0	4
Garlic mushrooms (not coated)	2 tbsp	50 g/2 oz	70	**140**	14.4	4
Garlic powder and purée – *see* Condiments, Jams & Ingredients, pages 170–72						
Guacamole, fresh	2 tbsp	50 g/2 oz	105	**210**	20.2	6
Guacamole, Mexican-style	2 tbsp	50 g/2 oz	102	**204**	20.4	5
Guacamole, reduced fat	2 tbsp	50 g/2 oz	63	**126**	10.1	5
Hash, vegetable and lentil	1 pack	200 g/7 oz	176	**88**	2.1	4
Hotpot, vegetable	1 bowl	300 g/11 oz	288	**96**	4.9	6
Kiev, vegetable	1	50 g/2 oz	105	**210**	13.4	3
Mornay, broccoli	1 pack	150 g/5 oz	140	**93**	6.2	5

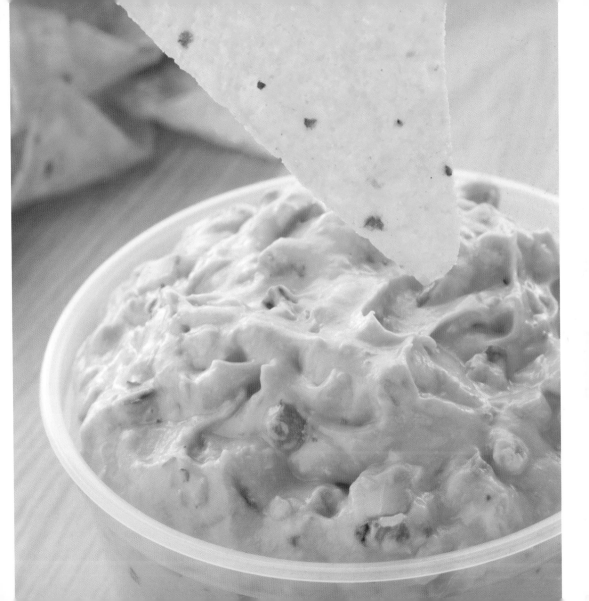

Counting Calories: Vegetables

	Typical portion	Typical portion size	Calories per portion	Calories per 100 g/ml	Fat per 100 g/ml	Health rating (1–10)
Mornay, spinach	1 pack	150 g/5 oz	135	**90**	6.9	5
Moussaka, aubergine and lentil	½ pack	200 g/7 oz	164	**82**	3.8	6
Moussaka, roasted vegetable	½ pack	200 g/7 oz	200	**100**	5.7	6
Nut roast	½ pack	160 g/5½ oz	533	**333**	23.5	6
Onion rings, breaded	5 rings	100 g/3½ oz	280	**280**	12.4	3
Onion rings, battered	5 rings	100 g/3½ oz	236	**236**	13.3	2
Pakora/bhajia, vegetable	1 pack	225 g/8 oz	528	**235**	14.7	4
Pancake, stuffed with vegetables	1	50 g/2 oz	118	**137**	7.6	5
Parmigiana, aubergine	3 tbsp	80 g/3 oz	76	**95**	5.3	5
Pease pudding	3 tbsp	80 g/3 oz	74	**93**	0.6	4
Pepper, stuffed	1 pepper	150 g/5 oz	144	**96**	5.0	7
Potato mash with bacon and cheese	3 tbsp	80 g/3 oz	101	**126**	6.4	4
Potato mash with cheese and onion	3 tbsp	80 g/3 oz	84	**105**	4.7	4
Pot. mash with savoy cabbage and spring onions	3 tbsp	80 g/3 oz	89	**111**	6.9	5
Potato mash with sweetcorn and flaked tuna	3 tbsp	80 g/3 oz	86	**107**	4.1	5
Potato mash with vegetables	3 tbsp	80 g/3 oz	50	**62**	1.0	5
Potato skins, cheese and bacon	3 tbsp	80 g/3 oz	176	**220**	12.0	5
Potato skins, cheese and ham	3 tbsp	80 g/3 oz	114	**143**	4.5	5
Potato skins, sour cream	3 tbsp	80 g/3 oz	164	**205**	11.9	5
Potato, baked jacket, with baked beans	1	250 g/9 oz	315	**126**	4.3	6
Potato, baked jacket, with Cheddar cheese	1	250 g/9 oz	436	**173**	9.0	5
Potato, baked jacket, with coleslaw	1	250 g/9 oz	375	**150**	8.2	5

	Typical portion	Typical portion size	Calories per portion	Calories per 100 g/ml	Fat per 100 g/ml	Health rating (1–10)
Potato, baked jacket, three-bean chilli	1	250 g/9 oz	295	**118**	4.3	6
Potatoes, dauphinoise	3 tbsp	80 g/3 oz	102	**127**	7.2	4
Quorn burgers, original style	1	50 g/2 oz	73	**146**	4.8	3
Quorn Cumberland sausage	1	50 g/2 oz	60	**120**	4.4	3
Quorn escalopes, creamy garlic and mushroom	1	120 g/4 oz	266	**222**	12.5	3
Quorn spaghetti bolognese	½ pack	200 g/7 oz	120	**60**	0.9	3
Quorn, bacon style, rashers	3 strips	38 g/1⅓ oz	74	**198**	15.5	3
Quorn, chilli	4 tbsp	100 g/3½ oz	81	**81**	4.2	3
Ratatouille	3 tbsp	80 g/3 oz	66	**82**	7.0	6
Ratatouille, retail	1 pack	225 g/8 oz	176	**78**	6.6	5
Ratatouille, roasted vegetable	3 tbsp	80 g/3 oz	36	**45**	1.0	6
Salad, baby leaf	1 pack	100 g/3½ oz	20	**20**	1.9	7
Salad, Caesar, bagged	1 bowl	135 g/4¾ oz	225	**167**	13.3	4
Salad, cheese, layered	1 pack	100 g/3½ oz	205	**205**	17.0	4
Salad, chicken	1 pack	100 g/3½ oz	139	**139**	3.6	6
Salad, chicken, Cajun	1 pack	100 g/3½ oz	143	**143**	3.3	5
Salad, egg and ham, with dressing	1 pack	100 g/3½ oz	70	**70**	3.5	5
Salad, Greek style	1 pack	100 g/3½ oz	43	**43**	2.2	5
Salad, green	1 bowl	150 g/5 oz	18	**12**	0.3	6
Salad, king prawn and new potato	1 pack	100 g/3½ oz	60	**60**	2.3	7
Salad, Mediterranean	1 pack	100 g/3½ oz	26	**26**	1.3	6
Salad, potato, with mayonnaise	2 tbsp	50 g/2 oz	144	**287**	26.5	5

Counting Calories: Vegetables

	Typical portion	Typical portion size	Calories per portion	Calories per 100 g/ml	Fat per 100 g/ml	Health rating (1–10)
Salad, three-bean	1 pack	100 g/3½ oz	104	**104**	2.3	7
Salad, tuna Niçoise	1 pack	100 g/3½ oz	105	**105**	2.0	6
Salad, Waldorf	1 pack	100 g/3½ oz	193	**193**	17.7	5
Samosa, vegetable	1	28 g/1 oz	61	**217**	9.3	3
Sauerkraut	2 tbsp	50 g/2 oz	5	**9**	0.0	3
Sausages, vegetarian	2	70 g/2½ oz	126	**179**	9.4	4
Shepherd's pie, vegetable	1 pack	225 g/8 oz	228	**101**	4.9	5
Soups – see Snacks, Confectionery & Desserts, page 222						
Stir-fry mix, vegetable, fried in vegetable oil	1 pack	225 g/8 oz	144	**64**	3.6	5
Tagliatelle, with vegetables	1 pack	225 g/8 oz	167	**74**	3.0	4
Tomato paste	1 tbsp	20 g/¾ oz	19	**96**	0.2	5
Tomato paste, sun-dried	1 tbsp	20 g/¾ oz	77	**385**	35.1	5
Tomato purée	1 tsp	5 g/⅙ oz	4	**76**	0.3	6
'Vegiballs', Swedish style	1	30 g/1 oz	58	**194**	9.5	4

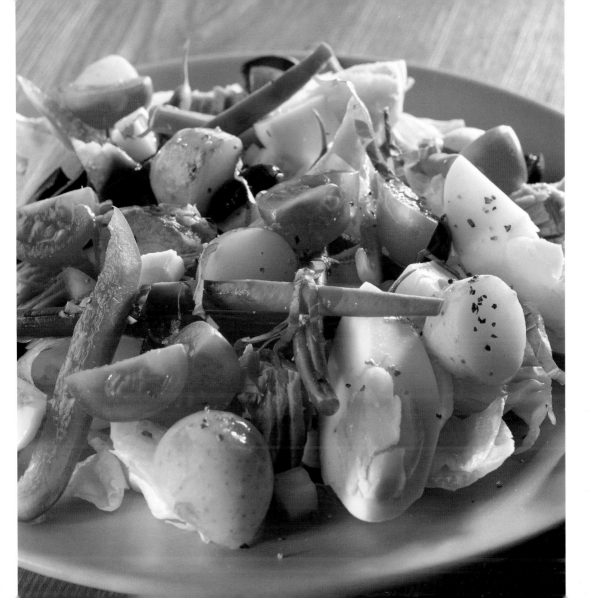

Fruit

	Typical portion	Typical portion size	Calories per portion	Calories per 100 g/ml	Fat per 100 g/ml	Health rating (1–10)
Tree and Shrub Fruit						
Ackee (brain fruit), canned, drained	2 tbsp	56 g/2 oz	85	**151**	15.2	7
Apple, cooking, raw, peeled	1	150 g/5 oz	53	**35**	0.1	8
Apple, cooking, stewed with sugar	2 tbsp	60 g/2 oz	45	**74**	0.1	4
Apple, cooking, stewed without sugar	2 tbsp	60 g/2 oz	20	**33**	0.1	7
Apple, eating, raw	1	120 g/4 oz	57	**47**	0.1	8
Apple, eating, raw, peeled	1	115 g/4 oz	52	**45**	0.1	7
Apricot, raw	2	50 g/2 oz	16	**31**	0.1	8
Apricot, dried, ready to eat	2	50 g/2 oz	79	**158**	0.6	8
Apricot, canned in juice	½ can	120 g/4 oz	41	**34**	0.1	8
Apricot, canned in syrup	½ can	120 g/4 oz	76	**63**	0.1	4
Avocado	½	75 g/3 oz	143	**190**	19.5	7
Banana	1	150 g/5 oz	143	**95**	0.3	8
Cherries, raw	1 handful	50 g/2 oz	24	**48**	0.1	9
Cherries, canned in syrup	2 tbsp	50 g/2 oz	31	**71**	0.0	4
Coconut, fresh – see Nuts, Seeds and Pulses, pages 77–78						
Damsons, raw	2	50 g/2 oz	19	**38**	0.0	8
Damsons, stewed with sugar	2 tbsp	56 g/2 oz	42	**74**	0.0	4
Dates, raw	3	50 g/2 oz	62	**124**	0.1	7

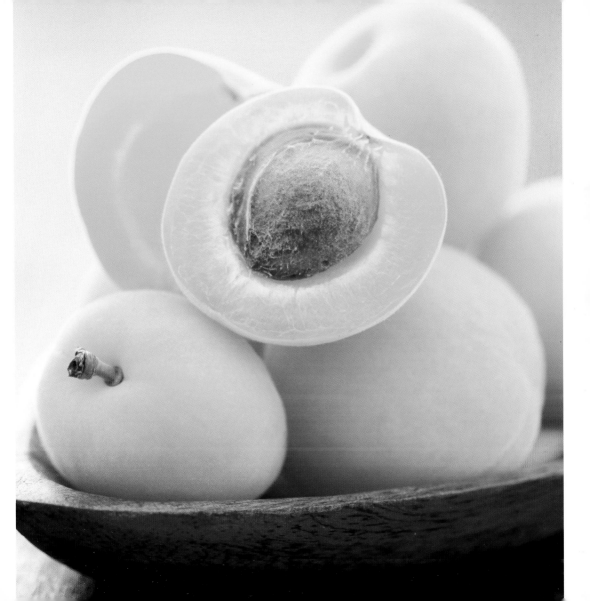

Counting Calories: Fruit

	Typical portion	Typical portion size	Calories per portion	Calories per 100 g/ml	Fat per 100 g/ml	Health rating (1–10)
Dragon fruit, raw, edible portion	1 pack	100 g/3½ oz	41	**41**	0.5	6
Figs, dried, ready to eat	2	50 g/2 oz	104	**209**	1.5	7
Guava, flesh only, raw	1	55 g/2 oz	37	**68**	1.0	8
Guava, canned in syrup	3 tbsp	80 g/3 oz	48	**60**	0.0	4
Lychees, raw	6	56 g/2 oz	33	**58**	0.1	7
Lychees, canned in syrup	½ can	102 g/3⅝ oz	70	**68**	0.0	4
Longans, canned in syrup	1 tbsp	28 g/1 oz	19	**67**	0.3	4
Loquats, raw	1	50 g/2 oz	14	**28**	0.2	7
Mango, ripe, raw	¼	50 g/2 oz	29	**57**	0.2	8
Mango in syrup	1 tbsp	20 g/¾ oz	16	**80**	0.0	4
Mango pieces in juice	1 tbsp	20 g/¾ oz	11	**56**	0.2	7
Mangosteen, raw, flesh only	1	80 g/3 oz	51	**63**	0.6	7
Mangosteen, canned in syrup, drained	1 tbsp	20 g/¾ oz	15	**73**	0.6	4
Medlar, raw, flesh only	1	28 g/1 oz	11	**40**	0.4	8
Nectarine	1	85 g/3 oz	34	**40**	0.1	8
Olives in brine	6	18 g/⅝ oz	18	**103**	11.0	5
Papaya, raw, flesh only	1	140 g/5 oz	37	**26**	0.1	8
Papaya pieces	1 handful	50 g/2 oz	178	**355**	0.0	8
Paw-paw, raw	1	80 g/3 oz	29	**36**	0.1	8
Paw-paw, canned in juice	½ can	125 g/4 oz	82	**65**	0.0	7
Peach, raw	1	85 g/3 oz	28	**33**	0.1	8
Peach, canned in juice	½ can	125 g/4 oz	49	**39**	0.0	7

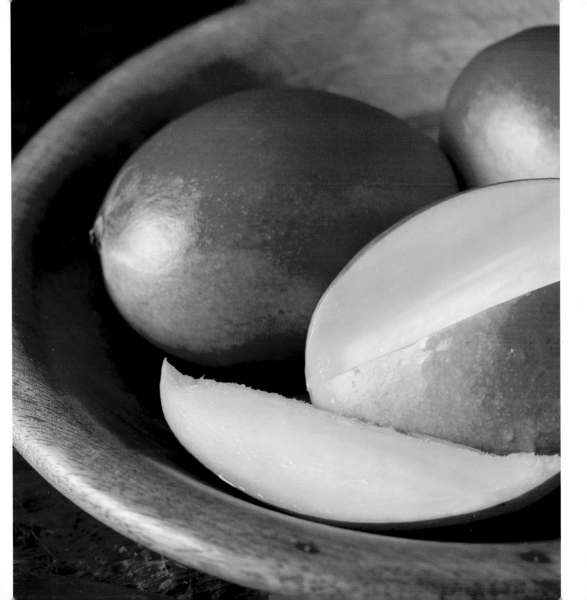

Counting Calories: Fruit

	Typical portion	Typical portion size	Calories per portion	Calories per 100 g/ml	Fat per 100 g/ml	Health rating (1–10)
Peach, canned in syrup	½ can	125 g/4 oz	68	**55**	0.0	4
Pear, raw	1	56 g/2 oz	23	**40**	0.1	8
Pear, raw, peeled	1	65 g/2½ oz	66	**41**	0.1	7
Pear, canned in juice	½ can	125 g/4 oz	83	**33**	0.0	7
Pear, canned in syrup	½ can	125 g/4 oz	63	**50**	0.0	4
Physalis (Cape gooseberry), raw, without husk	5	30 g/1 oz	16	**53**	0.7	7
Pineapple, raw	1 slice	56 g/2 oz	23	**41**	0.2	8
Pineapple, canned in juice	½ can	120 g/4 oz	57	**47**	0.0	8
Pineapple, canned in syrup	½ can	120 g/4 oz	77	**64**	0.0	4
Plums, raw	2	50 g/2 oz	18	**36**	0.1	8
Plums, stewed with sugar	2 tbsp	56 g/2 oz	57	**79**	0.1	4
Plums, canned in syrup	½ can	125 g/4 oz	74	**59**	0.0	4
Prunes, canned in juice	½ can	125 g/4 oz	99	**79**	0.2	7
Prunes, canned in syrup	½ can	105 g/3¾ oz	95	**90**	0.2	4
Prunes, dried, ready to eat	⅓ pack	75 g/3 oz	106	**141**	0.4	7
Quince	1	90 g/3¼ oz	23	**26**	0.1	6
Rhubarb, raw	n/a	n/a	n/a	**7**	0.1	7
Rhubarb, stewed with sugar	2 tbsp	56 g/2 oz	27	**48**	0.1	4
Rhubarb, canned in syrup	½ can	125 g/4 oz	39	**31**	0.0	4
Sharon fruit	1	20 g/¾ oz	15	**73**	0.0	6

Citrus Fruit

Clementine, raw without peel	1	46 g/1⅝ oz	22	**47**	0.1	7

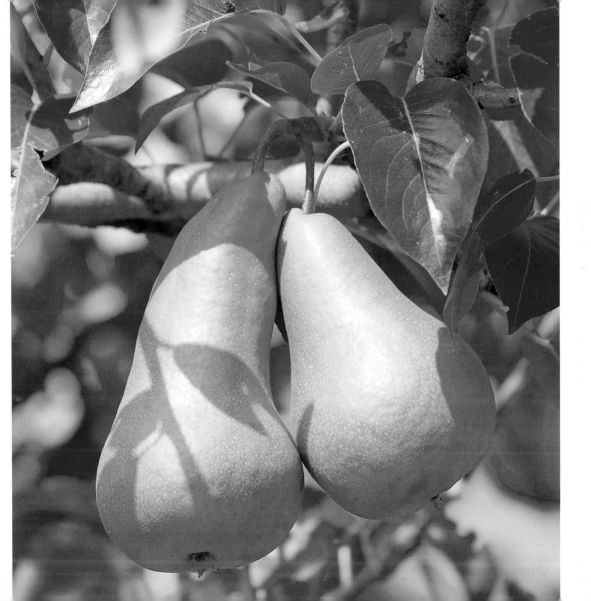

Counting Calories: Fruit

	Typical portion	Typical portion size	Calories per portion	Calories per 100 g/ml	Fat per 100 g/ml	Health rating (1–10)
Grapefruit, raw	½	80 g/3 oz	24	**30**	0.1	7
Grapefruit, canned in juice	½ can	125 g/4 oz	38	**30**	0.0	7
Grapefruit, canned in syrup	½ can	125 g/4 oz	75	**60**	0.0	4
Kumquat, raw	1	20 g/¾ oz	9	**43**	0.5	7
Kumquat, canned in syrup	1	20 g/¾ oz	28	**138**	0.5	4
Lemon peel	n/a	n/a	n/a	**19**	0.3	7
Lemon, whole, without pips	n/a	n/a	n/a	**19**	0.3	7
Lime	n/a	n/a	n/a	**19**	0.3	7
Mandarin orange, canned in juice	¼ can	102 g/3⅗ oz	33	**32**	0.0	7
Mandarin orange, canned in syrup	¼ can	102 g/3⅗ oz	54	**52**	0.0	4
Orange	1	85 g/3 oz	32	**37**	0.1	7
Pomelo, fresh, raw	½	100 g/3½ oz	38	**38**	0.0	7
Satsuma, flesh only	1	56 g/2 oz	20	**36**	0.1	7
Tangerine	1	50 g/2 oz	18	**35**	0.1	7

Berries and Vine Fruits

	Typical portion	Typical portion size	Calories per portion	Calories per 100 g/ml	Fat per 100 g/ml	Health rating (1–10)
Blackberries, raw	1 handful	50 g/2 oz	13	**25**	0.2	9
Blackberries, stewed with sugar	2 tbsp	56 g/2 oz	32	**56**	0.2	4
Blackcurrants, raw	1 handful	50 g/2 oz	14	**28**	0.0	9
Blackcurrants, stewed with sugar	2 tbsp	56 g/2 oz	33	**58**	0.0	4
Boysenberries, canned in syrup	1 handful	50 g/2 oz	44	**88**	0.1	4
Blueberries	1 handful	50 g/2 oz	28	**57**	0.3	9
Elderberries	1 handful	50 g/2 oz	18	**35**	0.5	8

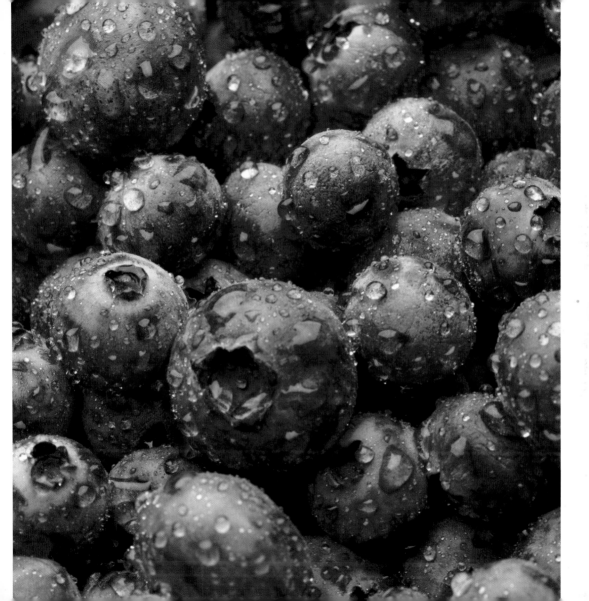

Counting Calories: Fruit

	Typical portion	Typical portion size	Calories per portion	Calories per 100 g/ml	Fat per 100 g/ml	Health rating (1–10)
Gooseberries, cooking, raw	2 tbsp	56 g/2 oz	11	**19**	0.4	8
Gooseberries, cooking, stewed with sugar	3 tbsp	56 g/2 oz	30	**54**	0.3	4
Grapes, green	1 handful	50 g/2 oz	31	**61**	0.1	8
Grapes, red	1 handful	50 g/2 oz	34	**67**	0.1	8
Kiwi fruit	1	60 g/2 oz	30	**49**	0.5	8
Loganberries, raw	1 handful	50 g/2 oz	9	**17**	0.0	8
Melon, cantaloupe type	1 slice	60 g/2 oz	12	**19**	0.1	7
Melon, galia	1 slice	60 g/2 oz	15	**24**	0.1	7
Melon, honeydew	1 slice	75 g/3 oz	21	**28**	0.1	7
Melon, watermelon	1 slice	75 g/3 oz	24	**31**	0.3	7
Mulberries, raw	1 handful	50 g/2 oz	18	**36**	0.0	8
Passion fruit	1	80 g/3 oz	29	**36**	0.4	8
Raspberries, raw	1 handful	50 g/2 oz	13	**25**	0.3	9
Raspberries, canned in syrup	½ can	105 g/3¾ oz	93	**88**	0.1	4
Strawberries, raw	6	50 g/2 oz	14	**27**	0.1	8
Strawberries, canned in syrup	½ can	105 g/3¾ oz	69	**65**	0.0	5

Dried Fruit

	Typical portion	Typical portion size	Calories per portion	Calories per 100 g/ml	Fat per 100 g/ml	Health rating (1–10)
Apple	1 pack	250 g/9 oz	554	**221**	0.3	7
Apricots	1 handful	50 g/2 oz	94	**188**	0.7	7
Banana	1 handful	50 g/2 oz	173	**346**	0.5	7
Cherries, glacé	n/a	n/a	n/a	**251**	0.0	3
Cranberries, sweetened	1 handful	50 g/2 oz	168	**335**	0.8	4

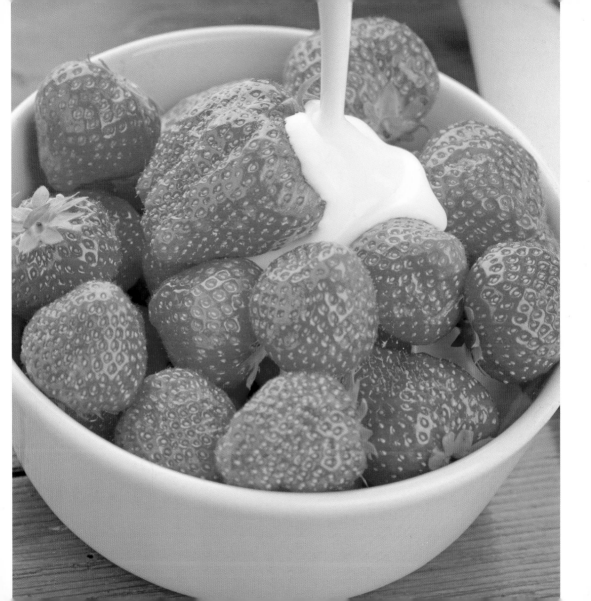

Counting Calories: Fruit

	Typical portion	Typical portion size	Calories per portion	Calories per 100 g/ml	Fat per 100 g/ml	Health rating (1–10)
Currants	1 handful	50 g/2 oz	133	**267**	0.4	7
Dates	4	50 g/2 oz	135	**270**	0.2	7
Exotic fruit, ready to eat	1 handful	50 g/2 oz	142	**284**	0.1	6
Figs	4	50 g/2 oz	114	**227**	1.6	7
Fruit salad	1 handful	50 g/2 oz	92	**183**	0.5	6
Goji berries	1 handful	50 g/2 oz	144	**287**	0.7	7
Mango	1 pack	100 g/3½ oz	347	**347**	1.0	7
Mix, Hawaiian	1 handful	50 g/2 oz	157	**314**	0.8	6
Mixed fruit, average	1 handful	50 g/2 oz	134	**268**	0.4	7
Mixed fruit (berries)	1 handful	50 g/2 oz	133	**265**	0.7	7
Mixed fruit (currants, sultanas, raisins, peel)	1 handful	50 g/2 oz	142	**283**	0.5	6
Mixed fruit and nuts (almonds, raisins, berries)	1 handful	50 g/2 oz	189	**377**	14.3	7
Mixed peel	n/a	n/a	n/a	**231**	0.9	4
Raisins	1 handful	50 g/2 oz	136	**272**	0.4	7
Sultanas	1 handful	50 g/2 oz	137	**275**	0.4	7

Mixed Fruit and Fruit Products

Compote, apple, strawberry and blackberry	3 tbsp	80 g/3 oz	52	**77**	0.1	6
Compote, apricot and prune	3 tbsp	80 g/3 oz	74	**92**	0.1	6
Compote, orchard fruits	3 tbsp	80 g/3 oz	50	**63**	0.1	6
Compote, strawberry and raspberry	3 tbsp	80 g/3 oz	72	**90**	0.1	6
Fruit cocktail, canned in juice	½ can	125 g/4 oz	37	**29**	0.0	7
Fruit cocktail, canned in syrup	½ can	125 g/4 oz	72	**57**	0.0	4

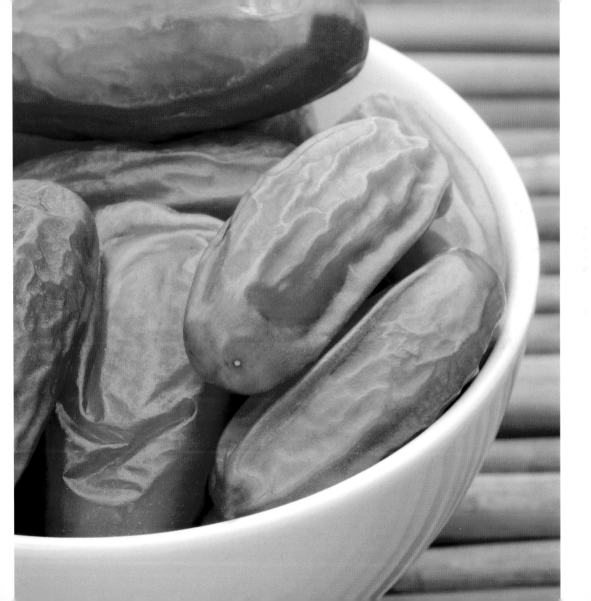

Counting Calories: Fruit

	Typical portion	Typical portion size	Calories per portion	Calories per 100 g/ml	Fat per 100 g/ml	Health rating (1–10)
Fruit salad, autumn	3 tbsp	75 g/3 oz	30	**40**	0.1	8
Fruit salad, average, retail	3 tbsp	75 g/3 oz	33	**44**	0.2	7
Fruit salad, berry	3 tbsp	75 g/3 oz	24	**31**	0.1	8
Fruit salad, citrus	3 tbsp	75 g/3 oz	27	**35**	0.1	7
Fruit salad, exotic	3 tbsp	75 g/3 oz	30	**42**	0.2	7
Fruit salad, fresh, home-made, unsweetened	3 tbsp	75 g/3 oz	42	**55**	0.1	8
Fruit salad, summer	3 tbsp	75 g/3 oz	30	**40**	0.2	8
Fruit salad, tropical	3 tbsp	75 g/3 oz	30	**41**	0.2	7
Mixed fruit in fruit juice	3 tbsp	80 g/3 oz	39	**49**	0.1	7
Mixed fruit in light syrup	3 tbsp	80 g/3 oz	46	**58**	0.1	5
Mixed fruit in syrup	3 tbsp	80 g/3 oz	60	**75**	0.1	4
Mixed fruit in very light syrup	3 tbsp	80 g/3 oz	24	**30**	0.0	5
Mixed fruit, no added sugar	3 tbsp	80 g/3 oz	40	**50**	0.1	7
Mixed fruit, tropical, in syrup	3 tbsp	80 g/3 oz	58	**73**	0.1	4
Pie filling, apricot	½ can	110 g/4 oz	87	**79**	0.1	3
Pie filling, black cherry	½ can	110 g/4 oz	121	**110**	0.1	3
Pie filling, Bramley apple	½ can	110 g/4 oz	94	**85**	0.1	3
Pie filling, mixed fruit	½ can	110 g/4 oz	85	**77**	0.0	3
Pie filling, red cherry	½ can	110 g/4 oz	108	**98**	0.0	3
Purée, apple and blueberry	1 pot	100 g/3½ oz	54	**54**	0.6	6
Purée, apple and peach	1 pot	100 g/3½ oz	49	**49**	0.3	6
Purée, banana, apple and peach	1 pot	100 g/3½ oz	68	**68**	0.4	6

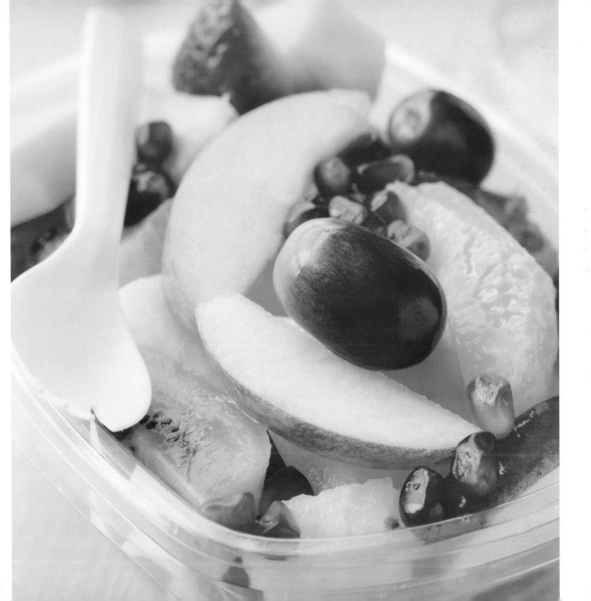

Condiments, Jams & Ingredients

	Typical portion	Typical portion size	Calories per portion	Calories per 100 g/ml	Fat per 100 g/ml	Health rating (1–10)
Dressings						
Dressing, blue cheese	1 dssp	10 g/¼ oz	46	**457**	46.3	3
Dressing, French, fat free	1 dssp	10 g/¼ oz	4	**39**	0.0	5
Dressing, thousand island	1 dssp	10 g/¼ oz	32	**323**	30.2	2
Mayonnaise	1 dssp	10 g/¼ oz	69	**691**	75.6	4
Mayonnaise, light	1 dssp	10 g/¼ oz	30	**298**	29.8	5
Mayonnaise, extra light	1 dssp	10 g/¼ oz	7	**73**	3.0	5
Mayonnaise, garlic	1 dssp	10 g/¼ oz	35	**346**	34.3	4
Mayonnaise, real	1 dssp	10 g/¼ oz	72	**722**	79.1	5
Salad cream	1 dssp	10 g/¼ oz	35	**348**	16.7	2
Salad cream, reduced calorie	1 dssp	10 g/¼ oz	20	**194**	9.4	2
Vinaigrette, balsamic	1 tbsp	15 ml/½ fl oz	12	**82**	2.7	2
Vinaigrette, French	1 tbsp	15 ml/½ fl oz	93	**620**	65.3	2
Vinaigrette, Portuguese	1 tbsp	15 ml/½ fl oz	61	**409**	44.0	2
Vinegar	1 tbsp	15 ml/½ fl oz	3	**22**	0.0	2
Vinegar, balsamic	1 tbsp	15 ml/½ fl oz	13	**88**	0.0	2
Vinegar, cider	1 tbsp	15 ml/½ fl oz	2	**14**	0.0	2
Vinegar, malt	1 tbsp	15 ml/½ fl oz	1	**4**	0.0	2
Vinegar, red wine	1 tbsp	15 ml/½ fl oz	3	**19**	0.0	2

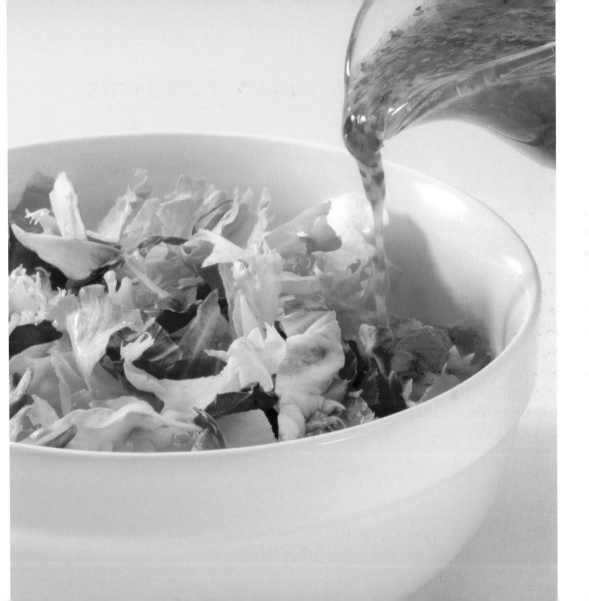

Counting Calories: Condiments, Jams & Ingredients

	Typical portion	Typical portion size	Calories per portion	Calories per 100 g/ml	Fat per 100 g/ml	Health rating (1–10)
Vinegar, white, rice	1 tbsp	15 ml/½ fl oz	1	**4**	0.0	2
Vinegar, white wine	1 tbsp	15 ml/½ fl oz	3	**19**	0.0	2

Sauces and Sauce Mixes

	Typical portion	Typical portion size	Calories per portion	Calories per 100 g/ml	Fat per 100 g/ml	Health rating (1–10)
Barbecue sauce	1 tsp	5 g/⅙ oz	5	**93**	0.1	2
Bolognese sauce, with meat	1 bowl	225 g/8 oz	362	**161**	11.6	4
Bread sauce, made with semi-skimmed milk	1 dssp	26 g/1 oz	27	**97**	2.5	4
Bread sauce, made with whole milk	1 dssp	26 g/1 oz	29	**110**	4.0	3
Brown sauce, sweet	1 tsp	5 g/⅙ oz	5	**98**	0.1	2
Cajun sauce for chicken	2 tbsp	75 g/3 oz	220	**294**	2.4	3
Casserole mix, beef	1 pack	43 g/1½ oz	111	**257**	1.0	2
Casserole mix, chicken	1 pack	43 g/1½ oz	56	**131**	4.3	2
Casserole mix, Moroccan lamb	1 pack	43 g/1½ oz	53	**124**	5.7	2
Casserole mix, sausage	1 pack	43 g/1½ oz	41	**96**	2.7	2
Cheese sauce packet mix, semi-skimmed milk	1 tbsp	50 g/2 oz	46	**91**	3.8	3
Cheese sauce packet mix, whole milk	1 tbsp	50 g/2 oz	55	**111**	6.0	2
Cheese sauce, made with semi-skimmed milk	1 tbsp	50 g/2 oz	90	**181**	12.8	4
Cheese sauce, made with whole milk	1 tbsp	50 g/2 oz	99	**198**	14.8	3
Cook-in sauces, packet	1 tbsp	50 g/2 oz	22	**43**	0.8	2
Curry paste, balti	1 tbsp	15 g/½ oz	58	**388**	34.0	3
Curry paste, bhuna	1 tbsp	15 g/½ oz	60	**397**	56.2	3
Curry paste, garam masala	1 tbsp	15 g/½ oz	61	**403**	35.4	3
Curry paste, hot	1 tbsp	15 g/½ oz	37	**245**	19.2	3

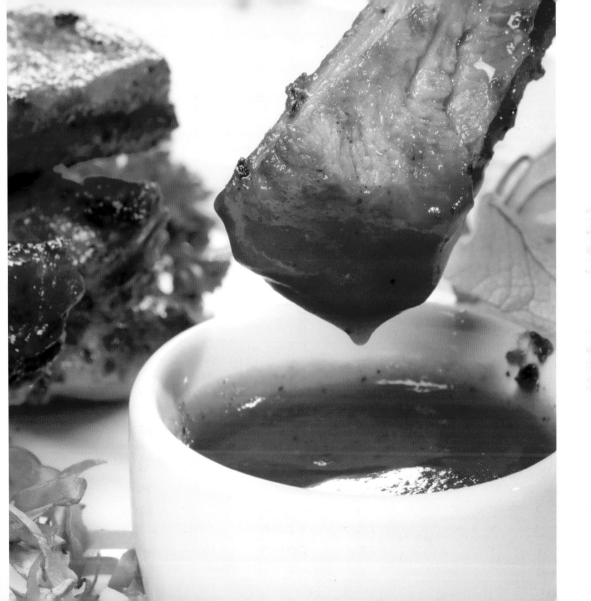

Counting Calories: Condiments, Jams & Ingredients

	Typical portion	Typical portion size	Calories per portion	Calories per 100 g/ml	Fat per 100 g/ml	Health rating (1–10)
Curry paste, jalfrezi	1 tbsp	15 g/½ oz	82	**549**	51.6	3
Curry paste, korma	1 tbsp	15 g/½ oz	62	**415**	39.0	3
Curry paste, madras	1 tbsp	15 g/½ oz	78	**520**	51.1	3
Curry paste, rogan josh	1 tbsp	15 g/½ oz	60	**397**	36.7	3
Curry paste, tandoori	1 tbsp	15 g/½ oz	34	**228**	15.8	3
Curry paste, Thai green	1 tbsp	15 g/½ oz	24	**156**	9.9	3
Curry paste, Thai red	1 tbsp	15 g/½ oz	23	**150**	10.8	3
Curry paste, tikka masala	1 tbsp	15 g/½ oz	29	**191**	15.4	3
Curry sauce, balti	¼ jar	125 g/4 oz	204	**163**	13.4	2
Curry sauce, canned	½ can	92 g/3¼ oz	78	**78**	19.5	2
Curry sauce, jalfrezi	¼ jar	125 g/4 oz	159	**127**	9.5	2
Curry sauce, korma	¼ jar	125 g/4 oz	305	**244**	17.0	2
Curry sauce, madras	¼ jar	125 g/4 oz	155	**124**	9.1	2
Curry sauce, masala	¼ jar	125 g/4 oz	101	**81**	4.9	2
Curry sauce, rogan josh	¼ jar	125 g/4 oz	243	**194**	15.8	2
Curry sauce, Thai green	¼ jar	125 g/4 oz	96	**77**	5.8	2
Curry sauce, tikka masala	¼ jar	125 g/4 oz	258	**206**	16.2	2
Curry sauce, vindaloo	¼ jar	125 g/4 oz	149	**119**	8.6	2
Horseradish sauce	1 tsp	5 g/⅙ oz	8	**153**	8.4	2
Ketchup, tomato	1 tbsp	15 g/½ oz	18	**120**	0.2	2
Ketchup, tomato, reduced sugar	1 tbsp	15 g/½ oz	13	**87**	1.2	3
Marinade, barbecue	2 tbsp	30 g/1 oz	45	**150**	0.2	4

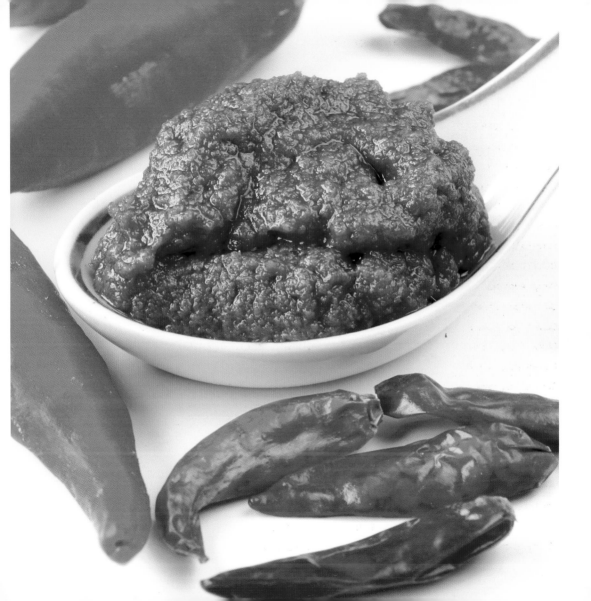

Counting Calories: Condiments, Jams & Ingredients

	Typical portion	Typical portion size	Calories per portion	Calories per 100 g/ml	Fat per 100 g/ml	Health rating (1–10)
Marinade, lemon and rosemary	2 tbsp	30 g/1 oz	44	**147**	13.0	4
Marinade, lime and coriander with piri-piri	2 tbsp	30 g/1 oz	55	**182**	16.6	4
Marinade, sticky barbecue	2 tbsp	30 g/1 oz	35	**115**	0.2	4
Marinade, tomato and herb	2 tbsp	30 g/1 oz	30	**100**	0.7	4
Marinade, white wine, garlic and pepper	2 tbsp	30 g/1 oz	30	**99**	0.7	3
Mint sauce	1 tsp	5 g/⅙ oz	5	**101**	0.0	2
Mustard, smooth	1 tsp	5 g/⅙ oz	7	**139**	8.2	2
Mustard, wholegrain	1 tsp	5 g/⅙ oz	7	**140**	10.2	2
Onion sauce, made with semi-skimmed milk	1 tbsp	50 g/2 oz	44	**88**	5.1	4
Onion sauce, made with whole milk	1 tbsp	50 g/2 oz	51	**101**	6.6	3
Passata Napolina	¼ jar	125 g/4 oz	31	**25**	0.1	5
Pasta sauce, arrabiata	½ pot	150 g/5 oz	54	**36**	1.0	5
Pasta sauce, bacon and mushroom	2 tbsp	75 g/3 oz	262	**349**	0.7	4
Pasta sauce, bolognese	½ pot	150 g/5 oz	120	**80**	4.1	5
Pasta sauce, carbonara	½ pot	150 g/5 oz	120	**80**	4.1	3
Pasta sauce, napoletana	½ pot	150 g/5 oz	126	**84**	5.6	5
Pasta sauce, roasted vegetable and olive	½ pot	150 g/5 oz	84	**56**	2.4	5
Pasta sauce, tomato-based	2 tbsp	75 g/3 oz	76	**47**	1.5	4
Pesto, chargrilled aubergine	1 tbsp	25 g/1 oz	85	**339**	34.9	3
Pesto, green	1 tbsp	25 g/1 oz	116	**462**	46.5	3
Pesto, roasted red peppers	1 tbsp	25 g/1 oz	60	**241**	22.8	3
Pesto, spinach and Parmesan	1 tbsp	25 g/1 oz	87	**349**	34.4	3

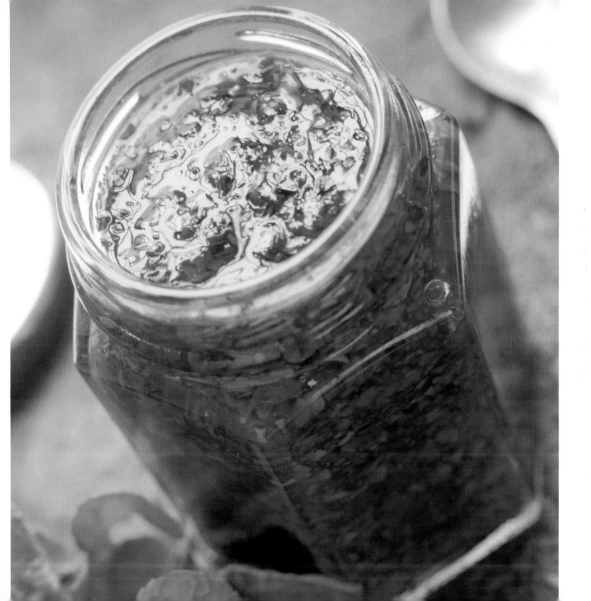

Counting Calories: Condiments, Jams & Ingredients

	Typical portion	Typical portion size	Calories per portion	Calories per 100 g/ml	Fat per 100 g/ml	Health rating (1–10)
Pesto, sun-dried tomato and wild rocket	1 tbsp	25 g/1 oz	106	**425**	43.5	3
Soy sauce	1 tsp	5 g/⅙ oz	2	**43**	0.0	1
Sweet and sour sauce, canned	½ can	92 g/3¼ oz	41	**44**	0.1	1
Sweet and sour sauce, takeaway	2 tbsp	75 g/3 oz	118	**157**	3.4	1
Tamarind paste	1 tbsp	15 g/½ oz	20	**133**	0.1	3
Tapenade paste, kalamata olive	1 tbsp	15 g/½ oz	43	**289**	30.6	3
Tartare sauce	1 tsp	5 g/⅙ oz	15	**299**	24.6	3
White sauce, savoury, with semi-skimmed milk	1 tbsp	50 g/2 oz	65	**130**	8.0	4
White sauce, savoury, with whole milk	1 tbsp	50 g/2 oz	75	**151**	10.3	3
Worcestershire sauce	1 tsp	5 g/⅙ oz	3	**65**	0.1	2
Dessert Sauces						
Chocolate	1 dssp	11 g/⅖ oz	35	**330**	9.4	1
Raspberry	1 dssp	11 g/⅖ oz	13	**120**	0.3	2
Toffee	1 dssp	11 g/⅖ oz	39	**355**	6.0	2
Stock and Savoury Extracts						
Bouillon, beef	1 tbsp	30 ml/1 fl oz	22	**73**	0.5	4
Bouillon, chicken	1 tbsp	30 ml/1 fl oz	23	**75**	3.0	4
Bouillon, fish	1 tbsp	30 ml/1 fl oz	21	**69**	0.3	4
Bouillon, vegetable	1 tbsp	30 ml/1 fl oz	30	**101**	0.3	6
Beef, fresh	1 tbsp	30 ml/1 fl oz	6	**18**	0.3	6
Chicken, fresh	1 tbsp	30 ml/1 fl oz	5	**16**	0.1	6
Fish, fresh	1 tbsp	30 ml/1 fl oz	3	**10**	0.0	6

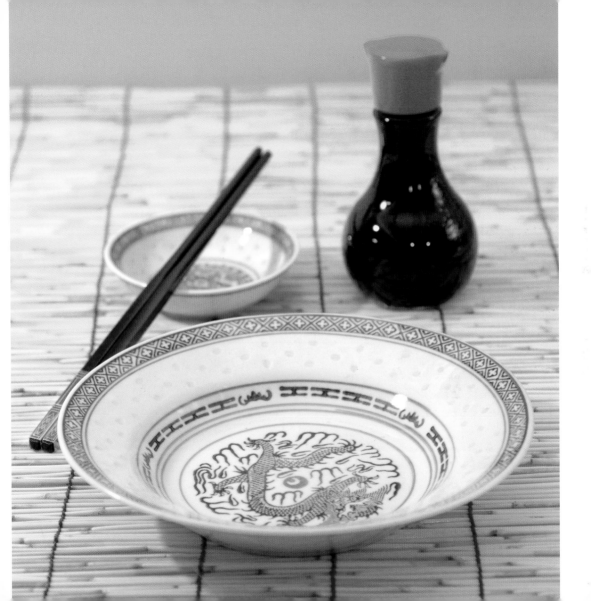

	Typical portion	Typical portion size	Calories per portion	Calories per 100 g/ml	Fat per 100 g/ml	Health rating (1–10)
Cubes, beef	1 cube	10 g/¼ oz	27	**265**	9.2	1
Cubes, chicken	1 cube	10 g/¼ oz	24	**237**	15.4	1
Cubes, vegetable	1 cube	10 g/¼ oz	25	**253**	17.3	1
Cubes, fish	1 cube	10 g/¼ oz	32	**321**	20.2	2
Cubes, ham	1 cube	10 g/¼ oz	31	**313**	18.7	2
Cubes, lamb	1 cube	10 g/¼ oz	30	**301**	21.2	2
Extract, yeast (e.g. Marmite)	1 tsp	9 g/¼ oz	21	**231**	0.1	5
Extract, beef (e.g. Bovril)	1 tsp	5 g/⅙ oz	1	**10**	4.1	5
Gravy						
Beef, fresh	3 tbsp	83 ml/3 fl oz	47	**56**	3.2	3
Beef, granules, dry	1 tbsp	16 g/½ oz	77	**480**	34.7	1
Chicken, granules, dry	1 tbsp	16 g/½ oz	47	**296**	4.9	1
Meat, granules	1 tbsp	16 g/½ oz	61	**384**	16.2	1
Vegetable, granules	1 tbsp	16 g/½ oz	51	**316**	4.9	1
Instant granules	1 tsp	5 g/⅙ oz	23	**462**	32.5	1
Instant granules, made up with water	3 tbsp	83 ml/3 fl oz	23	**34**	2.4	1
Cubes, beef	1 cube	10 g/¼ oz	33	**347**	25.3	2
Cubes, chicken	1 cube	10 g/¼ oz	30	**301**	18.5	2
Cubes, vegetable	1 cube	10 g/¼ oz	33	**330**	24.0	2
Chutneys and Pickles						
Chutney, apple	1 dssp	10 g/¼ oz	19	**190**	0.2	3
Chutney, Bengal, hot	1 dssp	10 g/¼ oz	20	**200**	0.3	2

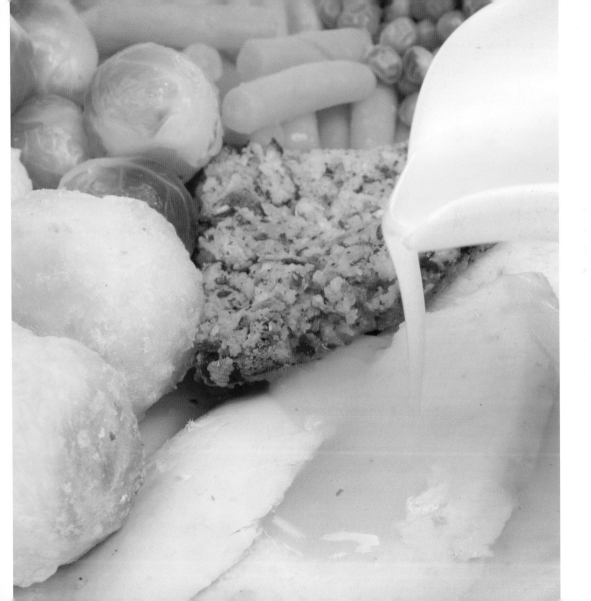

Counting Calories: Condiments, Jams & Ingredients

	Typical portion	Typical portion size	Calories per portion	Calories per 100 g/ml	Fat per 100 g/ml	Health rating (1–10)
Chutney, mango and lime	1 dssp	10 g/¼ oz	20	**206**	0.3	3
Chutney, mango, hot	1 dssp	10 g/¼ oz	26	**258**	0.2	3
Chutney, mango, sweet	1 dssp	10 g/¼ oz	19	**189**	0.1	3
Chutney, spiced fruit	1 dssp	10 g/¼ oz	15	**143**	0.1	2
Chutney, tomato	1 dssp	10 g/¼ oz	13	**128**	0.2	3
Piccalilli	1 dssp	10 g/¼ oz	8	**84**	0.5	3
Piccalilli, sweet	1 dssp	10 g/¼ oz	11	**112**	0.2	3
Pickle, chilli	1 dssp	10 g/¼ oz	13	**130**	0.7	3
Pickle, lime, hot	1 dssp	10 g/¼ oz	12	**123**	10.0	3
Pickle, lime, oily	1 dssp	10 g/¼ oz	18	**178**	15.5	3
Pickle, sweet	1 dssp	10 g/¼ oz	14	**141**	0.1	2
Relish, burger; chilli and tomato	1 tsp	5 g/⅙ oz	6	**114**	0.1	2
Relish, corn, cucumber and onion	1 tsp	5 g/⅙ oz	6	**119**	0.3	2

Dips

Blue cheese	1 dssp	20 g/¾ oz	68	**337**	34.5	2
Cheddar and onion	1 dssp	20 g/¾ oz	20	**100**	4.6	2
Cheese and chive	1 dssp	20 g/¾ oz	78	**390**	40.4	2
Cheese and chive, half fat	1 dssp	20 g/¾ oz	35	**172**	12.7	3
Chilli	1 dssp	20 g/¾ oz	59	**295**	0.2	3
Mozzarella	1 dssp	20 g/¾ oz	68	**337**	34.5	3
Mustard and honey	1 dssp	20 g/¾ oz	71	**356**	36.3	3
Nacho cheese	1 dssp	20 g/¾ oz	54	**270**	23.7	3

	Typical portion	Typical portion size	Calories per portion	Calories per 100 g/ml	Fat per 100 g/ml	Health rating (1–10)
Onion and garlic	1 dssp	20 g/¾ oz	96	**480**	50.4	3
Smoked salmon and dill	1 dssp	20 g/¾ oz	88	**439**	44.7	3
Smoked salmon and dill, reduced fat	1 dssp	20 g/¾ oz	43	**217**	19.7	3
Sour-cream based	1 dssp	20 g/¾ oz	72	**360**	37.0	3
Tangy barbecue	1 dssp	20 g/¾ oz	1	**100**	0.6	3
Thousand Island	1 dssp	20 g/¾ oz	49	**245**	22.2	3
Yogurt, cucumber and dill	1 dssp	20 g/¾ oz	24	**121**	7.2	3

Jams, Preserves and Spreads

	Typical portion	Typical portion size	Calories per portion	Calories per 100 g/ml	Fat per 100 g/ml	Health rating (1–10)
Apricot conserve	1 tsp	7 g/¼ oz	16	**244**	0.2	2
Apricot conserve, reduced sugar	1 tsp	7 g/¼ oz	13	**184**	0.2	2
Blackberry jelly	1 tsp	7 g/¼ oz	13	**182**	0.2	2
Blackcurrant jelly	1 tsp	7 g/¼ oz	15	**232**	0.2	2
Chocolate spread	1 tbsp	15 g/½ oz	85	**569**	37.6	1
Honey, clear, Canadian clover	1 tbsp	15 g/½ oz	51	**339**	0.1	3
Honey, clear, pure	1 tbsp	15 g/½ oz	47	**314**	0.0	3
Honey, clear, Scottish heather	1 tbsp	15 g/½ oz	46	**307**	0.0	3
Honey, set, pure	1 tbsp	15 g/½ oz	47	**312**	0.0	3
Lemon curd	1 tbsp	15 g/½ oz	44	**294**	4.7	3
Marmalade, grapefruit	1 tbsp	15 g/½ oz	39	**261**	0.0	2
Marmalade, lemon	1 tbsp	15 g/½ oz	37	**247**	0.0	2
Marmalade, lemon and lime	1 tbsp	15 g/½ oz	40	**267**	0.1	2
Marmalade, lime	1 tbsp	15 g/½ oz	39	**261**	0.1	2

	Typical portion	Typical portion size	Calories per portion	Calories per 100 g/ml	Fat per 100 g/ml	Health rating (1–10)
Marmalade, orange, reduced sugar	1 tbsp	15 g/½ oz	26	**170**	0.1	2
Marmalade, orange, thick cut with Drambuie	1 tbsp	15 g/½ oz	49	**329**	0.0	2
Marmalade, orange, with shred	1 tbsp	15 g/½ oz	40	**263**	0.0	2
Marmalade, three fruit	1 tbsp	15 g/½ oz	39	**262**	0.1	2
Mixed fruit jam	1 tsp	7 g/¼ oz	17	**252**	0.2	2
Mixed fruit jam, reduced sugar	1 tsp	7 g/¼ oz	13	**180**	0.3	2
Raspberry jelly	1 tsp	7 g/¼ oz	16	**236**	0.2	2
Redcurrant jelly	1 tsp	7 g/¼ oz	15	**234**	0.2	2
Strawberry jelly	1 tsp	7 g/¼ oz	15	**234**	0.2	2
Spices and Herbs						
Cinnamon	1 tsp	3 g/⅑ oz	8	**261**	3.2	4
Coriander, fresh	1 dssp	10 g/¼ oz	3	**23**	0.5	6
Coriander, dried	1 tsp	5 g/⅙ oz	14	**279**	4.8	6
Cumin seeds	1 tsp	5 g/⅙ oz	19	**375**	22.7	5
Curry leaves, fresh	1 tbsp	27 g/1 oz	27	**97**	1.3	5
Curry powder	1 tbsp	2 g/²⁄₂₈ oz	6	**325**	13.8	3
Dill, dried	1 tsp	15 g/½ oz	38	**253**	4.4	4
Dill, fresh, chopped	1 tbsp	15 g/½ oz	4	**25**	0.8	6
Fenugreek leaves, raw, fresh	1 tbsp	3 g/⅑ oz	1	**35**	0.2	5
Five-spice powder	1 tsp	2 g/²⁄₂₈ oz	4	**172**	8.6	3
Garam masala	1 tbsp	15 g/½ oz	57	**379**	15.1	3
Garlic powder	1 tsp	3 g/⅑ oz	7	**246**	1.2	6

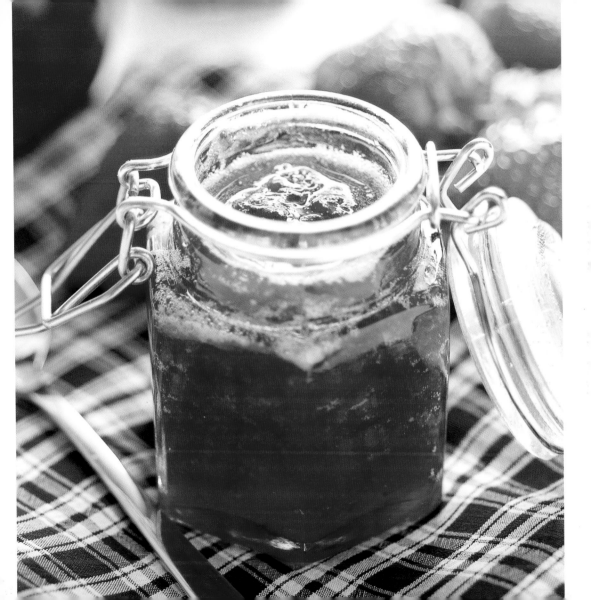

Counting Calories: Condiments, Jams & Ingredients

	Typical portion	Typical portion size	Calories per portion	Calories per 100 g/ml	Fat per 100 g/ml	Health rating (1–10)
Garlic purée	1 tbsp	15 g/½ oz	57	**380**	33.6	5
Ginger, ground	1 tsp	3 g/⅑ oz	8	**258**	3.3	5
Ginger, root, raw	1 tsp	3 g/⅑ oz	3	**86**	0.8	5
Horseradish, prepared	1 tsp	5 g/⅙ oz	3	**62**	0.3	5
Marjoram, dried	1 tsp	5 g/⅙ oz	14	**271**	7.0	5
Mint, dried	1 tsp	5 g/⅙ oz	14	**279**	4.6	5
Mint, fresh	1 tbsp	5 g/⅙ oz	2	**43**	0.7	4
Mixed herbs, average, dried	1 tsp	5 g/⅙ oz	13	**260**	8.5	4
Mixed herbs, de Provence, dried	1 tsp	5 g/⅙ oz	18	**364**	5.8	4
Nutmeg, ground	1 tsp	5 g/⅙ oz	26	**525**	36.3	5
Oregano, dried	1 tsp	5 g/⅙ oz	15	**306**	10.3	5
Oregano, fresh	1 tbsp	5 g/⅙ oz	4	**66**	2.0	5
Paprika	1 tsp	5 g/⅙ oz	14	**289**	13.0	5
Parsley, dried	1 tsp	5 g/⅙ oz	9	**181**	7.0	5
Parsley, fresh	1 tbsp	5 g/⅙ oz	2	**34**	1.3	3
Pepper, black, freshly ground	1 tsp	2 g/²⁄₂₈ oz	5	**255**	3.3	3
Pepper, cayenne, ground	1 tsp	2 g/²⁄₂₈ oz	6	**318**	17.3	3
Pepper, white	1 tsp	2 g/²⁄₂₈ oz	6	**296**	2.1	3
Rosemary, dried	1 tsp	2 g/²⁄₂₈ oz	7	**331**	15.2	5
Rosemary, fresh	1 tbsp	5 g/⅙ oz	5	**99**	4.4	5
Saffron	1 tsp	1 g/¹⁄₂₈ oz	2	**310**	5.9	5
Sage, dried, ground	1 tsp	2 g/²⁄₂₈ oz	6	**315**	12.7	6

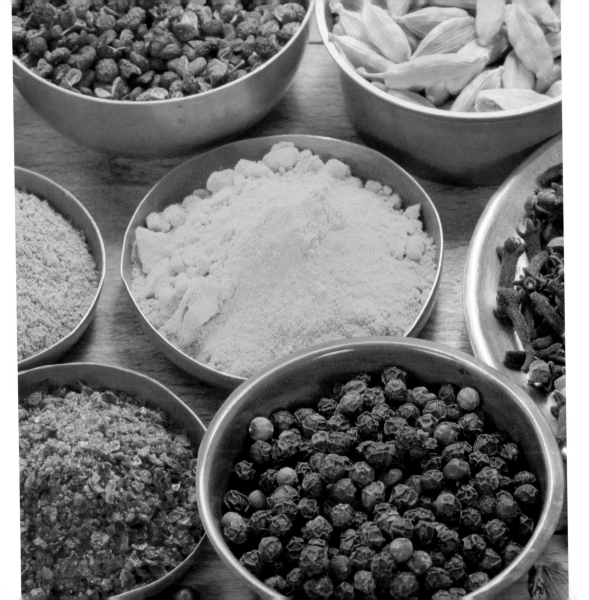

	Typical portion	Typical portion size	Calories per portion	Calories per 100 g/ml	Fat per 100 g/ml	Health rating (1–10)
Sage, fresh	1 tbsp	5 g/⅙ oz	7	**119**	4.6	6
Seasoning, aromatic	2 tbsp	30 g/1 oz	49	**164**	3.6	2
Sushi (powder)	2 tbsp	30 g/1 oz	50	**167**	3.3	2
Tarragon, dried	1 tsp	2 g/²⁄₂₈ oz	5	**295**	7.2	5
Tarragon, fresh	1 tbsp	10 g/¼ oz	5	**49**	1.1	5
Thyme, dried, ground	1 tsp	2 g/²⁄₂₈ oz	6	**276**	7.4	5
Thyme, fresh	1 tbsp	10 g/¼ oz	10	**95**	2.5	5
Seasoning cubes for rice, pilaf	1	10 g/¼ oz	30	**305**	22.6	2
Seasoning cubes for stir-fry	1	10 g/¼ oz	41	**414**	30.6	2
Store Cupboard						
Baking powder	1 tsp	5 g/⅙ oz	8	**163**	0.0	1
Batter mix	1 tbsp	20 g/¾ oz	40	**200**	1.5	2
Cake mix, carrot cake	¼ pack	75 g/3 oz	301	**403**	6.7	2
Cake mix, cheesecake	¼ pack	75 g/3 oz	201	**268**	12.0	2
Cake mix, chocolate brownie	¼ pack	75 g/3 oz	225	**299**	7.1	2
Cream of Tartar	1 tsp	3 g/⅑ oz	8	**258**	0.0	1
Crumble mix	¼ pack	75 g/3 oz	330	**441**	16.3	2
Extract, almond	1 tbsp	13 g/½ oz	37	**288**	0.1	1
Extract, vanilla	1 tbsp	13 g/½ oz	37	**288**	0.1	1
Gelatine	1 tsp	5 g/⅙ oz	17	**338**	0.0	1
Molasses	1 tbsp	20 g/¾ oz	53	**266**	0.1	1
Muffin mix	1 pack	50 g/2 oz	217	**433**	16.7	2

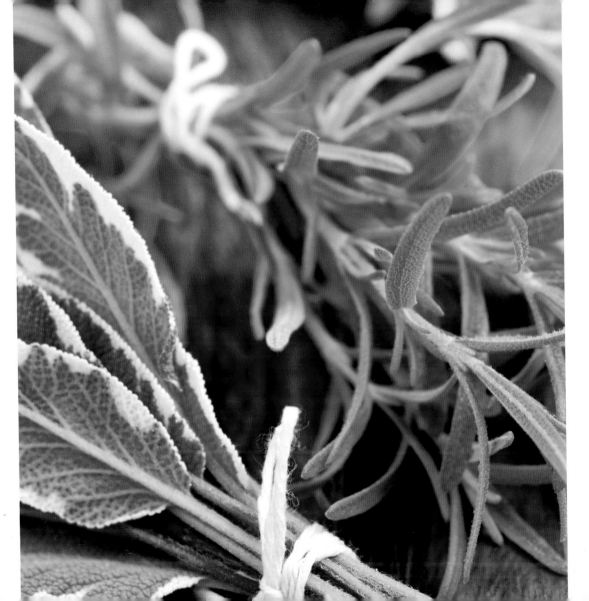

Counting Calories: Condiments, Jams & Ingredients

	Typical portion	Typical portion size	Calories per portion	Calories per 100 g/ml	Fat per 100 g/ml	Health rating (1–10)
Nachos kit	½ pack	260 g/9 oz	598	**230**	10.0	2
Pancake mix	1 pancake	38 g/1⅓ oz	89	**235**	13.1	2
Pizza base mix	1 pack	75 g/3 oz	266	**355**	3.8	2
Salt	1 tsp	5 g/⅙ oz	0	**0**	0.0	1
Scone mix, fruit	1 pack	50 g/2 oz	151	**301**	5.0	2
Stuffing mix, dried	¼ pack	30 g/1 oz	100	**338**	5.2	2
Stuffing, sage and onion	¼ pack	30 g/1 oz	81	**269**	15.1	2
Sugar, brown, soft	1 tsp	4 g/⅐ oz	15	**382**	0.0	1
Sugar, caster	1 tsp	4 g/⅐ oz	16	**399**	0.0	1
Sugar, demerara	1 tsp	5 g/⅙ oz	18	**367**	0.0	1
Sugar, for jam making	1 tsp	28 g/1 oz	111	**398**	0.0	1
Sugar, fructose	1 tsp	4 g/⅐ oz	16	**400**	0.0	1
Sugar, golden/unrefined	1 tsp	4 g/⅐ oz	18	**399**	0.0	1
Sugar, icing	1 tsp	4 g/⅐ oz	16	**394**	0.0	1
Sugar, white, granulated	1 tsp	5 g/⅙ oz	20	**397**	0.0	1
Sweetener	1 tsp	1 g/1/28 oz	4	**392**	0.0	1
Syrup, corn	1 tbsp	20 g/¾ oz	56	**282**	0.0	1
Syrup, golden	1 tbsp	20 g/¾ oz	61	**304**	0.0	1
Syrup, maple	1 tbsp	20 g/¾ oz	52	**262**	0.2	1
Treacle, black	1 tbsp	20 g/¾ oz	51	**257**	0.0	1
Yeast, baker's, compressed	1 tsp	5 g/⅙ oz	3	**53**	0.4	1
Yeast, baker's, dried	1 tsp	5 g/⅙ oz	7	**169**	1.5	1

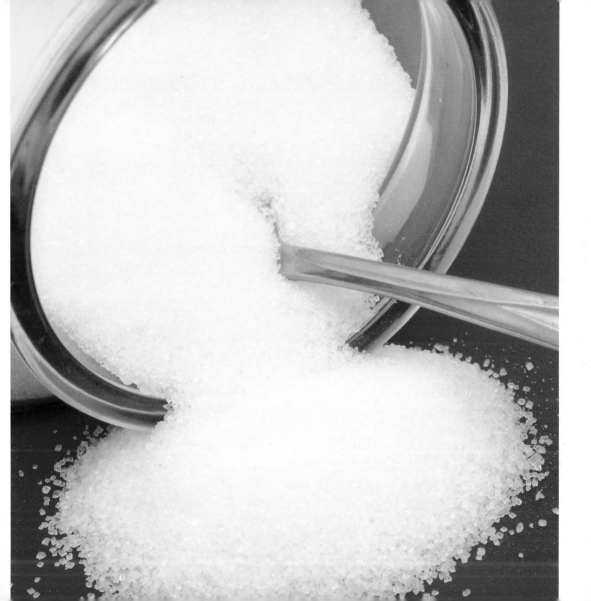

Breads & Baked Products

	Typical portion	Typical portion size	Calories per portion	Calories per 100 g/ml	Fat per 100 g/ml	Health rating (1–10)
Breads and Scones						
White, batch	1 slice	42 g/1½ oz	98	**233**	2.1	4
White, farmhouse	1 slice	44 g/1 5/9 oz	99	**226**	1.6	4
White, thin sliced	1 slice	29 g/1 oz	66	**228**	1.5	4
White, medium sliced	1 slice	36 g/1¼ oz	78	**216**	1.9	4
White, thick sliced	1 slice	44 g/1 5/9 oz	95	**216**	1.9	4
White, toasted	1 slice	33 g/1⅙ oz	87	**265**	1.6	4
White, wheat and gluten free	1 slice	33 g/1⅙ oz	75	**227**	8.6	4
Brown, thin sliced	1 slice	29 g/1 oz	65	**225**	1.9	6
Brown, medium sliced	1 slice	34 g/1⅕ oz	74	**218**	2.0	6
Brown, thick sliced	1 slice	50 g/2 oz	109	**219**	2.5	6
Brown, medium sliced, toasted	1 slice	24 g/6/7 oz	65	**272**	2.1	6
Brown, multigrain, wheat and gluten free	1 slice	33 g/1⅙ oz	76	**229**	5.1	7
Brown, premium malted	1 slice	43 g/1½ oz	93	**217**	2.4	6
Wholemeal, medium sliced	1 slice	40 g/1⅖ oz	86	**216**	2.7	7
Wholemeal, thick sliced	1 slice	48 g/1⅔ oz	102	**213**	2.6	7
Wholemeal, medium sliced, toasted	1 slice	26 g/1 oz	58	**224**	2.2	7
Granary, average	1 slice	35 g/1¼ oz	82	**235**	2.7	7
Bagel, plain	1	85 g/3¼ oz	232	**273**	1.8	3

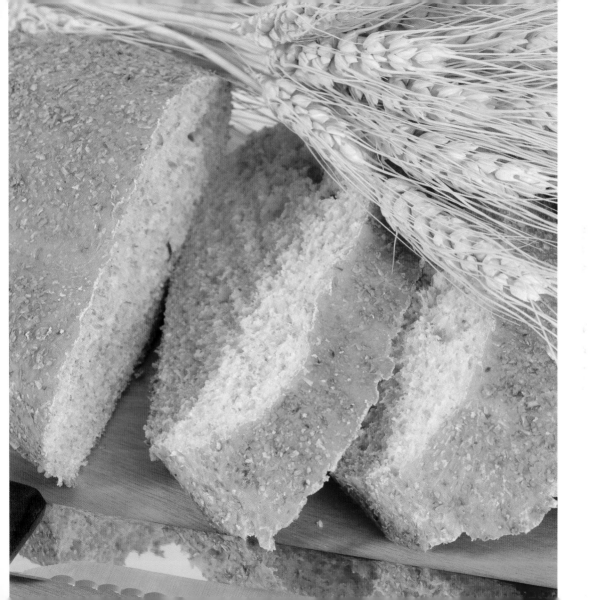

Counting Calories: Breads & Baked Products

	Typical portion	Typical portion size	Calories per portion	Calories per 100 g/ml	Fat per 100 g/ml	Health rating (1–10)
Bagel, wholemeal	1	85 g/3¼ oz	216	**254**	1.7	5
Baguette, garlic	½	85 g/3 oz	342	**403**	19.2	3
Bruschetta	1	75 g/3 oz	367	**489**	25.1	4
Burger bun/bap, white	1	56 g/2 oz	154	**275**	5.2	4
Challah	1 slice	50 g/2 oz	143	**286**	7.1	2
Challah, cheese onion and garlic	¼	112 g/4 oz	326	**290**	13.0	2
Chapatti, brown	3	42 g/1½ oz	128	**305**	8.0	5
Chapatti, made with fat	1	60 g/2 oz	197	**328**	12.8	3
Chapatti, made without fat	2	55 g/2 oz	111	**202**	1.0	3
Chapatti, wholemeal	4	42 g/1½ oz	130	**310**	9.5	6
Ciabatta, black olive	¼	65 g/2½ oz	167	**257**	3.8	4
Ciabatta, garlic and herb	¼	65 g/2½ oz	150	**230**	2.4	4
Ciabatta, plain	¼	65 g/2½ oz	156	**240**	3.9	4
Ciabatta, ready to bake	½	66 g/2½ oz	172	**260**	3.7	4
Ciabatta, sun-dried tomato and basil	¼	65 g/2½ oz	167	**257**	5.7	4
Cottage loaf	1 slice	67 g/2½ oz	155	**232**	1.3	4
Croissant	1	44 g/1 5/9 oz	151	**343**	14.8	3
Croissant, cheese and ham	1	65 g/2½ oz	249	**383**	24.5	3
Croissant, reduced fat	1	44 g/1 5/9 oz	173	**393**	17.5	3
Crumpet	1	46 g/1⅝ oz	86	**186**	0.7	3
Crumpet, fruit	1	73 g/2 4/7 oz	161	**220**	2.3	3
Crumpet, toasted	1	40 g/1½ oz	80	**199**	1.0	3

	Typical portion	Typical portion size	Calories per portion	Calories per 100 g/ml	Fat per 100 g/ml	Health rating (1–10)
English muffin, white	1	57 g/2 oz	120	**211**	1.8	3
Flatbread (focaccia)	¼	70 g/2½ oz	195	**279**	5.9	4
Flatbread, garlic and herb	¼	68 g/2½ oz	201	**297**	9.3	4
French baguette	4 cm slice	150 g/5 oz	360	**240**	1.2	4
Malt loaf, fruity	1 slice	42 g/1½ oz	130	**310**	2.0	5
Malted brown loaf	1 slice	44 g/1⅗ oz	111	**249**	2.0	6
Melba toast	1 slice	3 g/⅛ oz	13	**396**	4.9	3
Multigrain loaf	1 slice	50 g/2 oz	117	**235**	2.9	7
Multigrain loaf, gluten free	1 slice	17 g/⅗ oz	39	**229**	5.0	7
Naan, garlic and coriander	1	140 g/5 oz	452	**323**	10.8	3
Naan, peshwari	1	130 g/4½ oz	338	**260**	5.6	3
Naan, plain	1	130 g/4½ oz	337	**259**	5.8	3
Pitta, white	1	56 g/2 oz	147	**262**	1.9	4
Pitta, wholemeal	1	56 g/2 oz	143	**255**	1.3	6
Roll, brown, crusty	1	50 g/2 oz	127	**255**	2.8	4
Roll, brown, finger	1	46 g/1⅝ oz	119	**259**	1.8	6
Roll, brown, soft	1	50 g/2 oz	134	**268**	3.8	6
Roll, granary	1	70 g/2½ oz	180	**257**	4.1	7
Roll, white, crusty	1	50 g/2 oz	131	**262**	2.2	4
Roll, white, soft	1	50 g/2 oz	127	**254**	2.6	4
Roll, wholemeal	1	45 g/1⅗ oz	108	**241**	2.9	7
Rye bread	1 slice	35 g/1¼ oz	77	**219**	1.7	7

	Typical portion	Typical portion size	Calories per portion	Calories per 100 g/ml	Fat per 100 g/ml	Health rating (1–10)
Scone, plain	1	40 g/1½ oz	146	**364**	14.8	3
Scone, all butter	1	50 g/2 oz	154	**308**	7.8	4
Scone, cheese	1	50 g/2 oz	179	**357**	18.6	4
Scone, with fresh cream and strawberry jam	1	50 g/2 oz	176	**352**	18.9	3
Scone, fruit	1	50 g/2 oz	163	**325**	8.2	5
Scone, wholemeal	1	50 g/2 oz	163	**325**	14.4	5
Scone, wholemeal fruit	1	50 g/2 oz	162	**324**	12.8	6
Soda bread	1 slice	35 g/1¼ oz	90	**258**	2.5	5
Wheatgerm bread	1 slice	30 g/1 oz	90	**300**	4.0	7

Sandwiches – *see* Snacks, Confectionery & Desserts, page 214

Biscuits, Cookies and Crackers

	Typical portion	Typical portion size	Calories per portion	Calories per 100 g/ml	Fat per 100 g/ml	Health rating (1–10)
All butter biscuits	1	10 g/¼ oz	44	**487**	23.0	2
All butter sultana cookies	1	16 g/⅔ oz	73	**455**	19.0	2
Almond fingers	1	28 g/1 oz	109	**390**	15.0	2
Almond thins	1	4 g/⅛ oz	13	**430**	9.0	2
Amaretti	1	4 g/⅛ oz	17	**433**	7.8	2
Apple strudel softies	1	23 g/⅚ oz	80	**348**	1.6	2
Biscotti, almond	1	30 g/1 oz	130	**433**	16.7	2
Biscotti, chocolate	1	30 g/1 oz	119	**398**	8.7	2
Bourbon creams	1	14 g/½ oz	69	**485**	21.0	2
Brandy snaps	1	12 g/⅜ oz	54	**452**	13.9	2
Butter puffs (crackers)	1	10 g/¼ oz	54	**523**	26.5	3

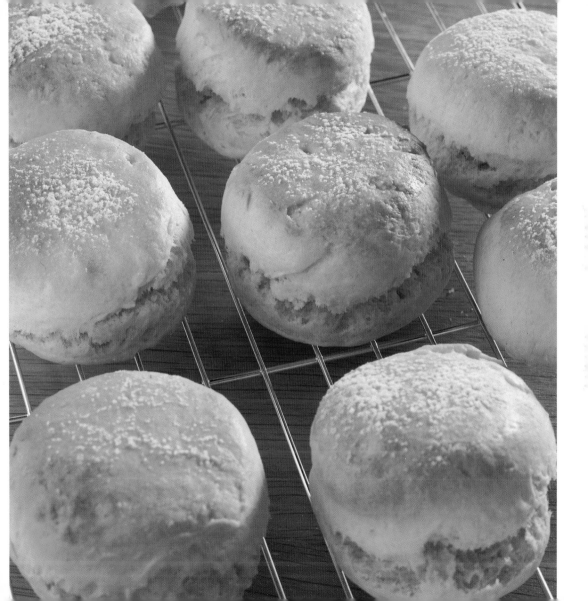

Counting Calories: Breads & Baked Products

	Typical portion	Typical portion size	Calories per portion	Calories per 100 g/ml	Fat per 100 g/ml	Health rating (1–10)
Cheddar crackers	1 packet	30 g/1 oz	155	**517**	30.0	3
Chocolate chip cookies	1	11 g/⅖ oz	56	**511**	23.9	2
Chocolate chip and hazelnut cookies	1	16 g/4/7 oz	88	**549**	33.3	2
Chocolate chip, double, cookies	1	22 g/⅞ oz	108	**490**	23.7	2
Chocolate fingers with caramel	1	25 g/1 oz	103	**410**	19.0	2
Chocolate fingers, milk	1	8 g/¼ oz	42	**526**	26.8	2
Chocolate fingers, plain	1	8 g/¼ oz	41	**508**	26.8	2
Chocolate fingers, white	1	8 g/¼ oz	43	**530**	28.2	2
Chocolate snack sandwich	1	26 g/1 oz	137	**525**	27.2	2
Crackers, cream	1	8 g/¼ oz	34	**431**	13.5	3
Crackers, wholemeal	1	14 g/½ oz	58	**414**	11.5	5
Crispbread, multigrain	1 slice	11 g/⅖ oz	36	**331**	5.2	4
Crispbread, rye	1 slice	10 g/¼ oz	32	**317**	1.7	4
Danish butter cookie	1	32 g/1⅛ oz	165	**516**	25.6	2
Digestive biscuits, chocolate	1	17 g/⅗ oz	84	**493**	24.1	3
Digestive biscuits, plain	1	14 g/½ oz	66	**471**	20.9	4
Fig rolls	1	18 g/⅝ oz	70	**377**	9.4	4
Florentines	1	8 g/¼ oz	40	**506**	30.8	3
Fruit shortcake	1	10 g/¼ oz	45	**445**	17.0	3
Garibaldi	1	10 g/¼ oz	40	**397**	10.4	3
Ginger crunch creams	1	14 g/½ oz	73	**518**	26.7	2
Ginger nuts	1	10 g/¼ oz	45	**450**	1.6	3

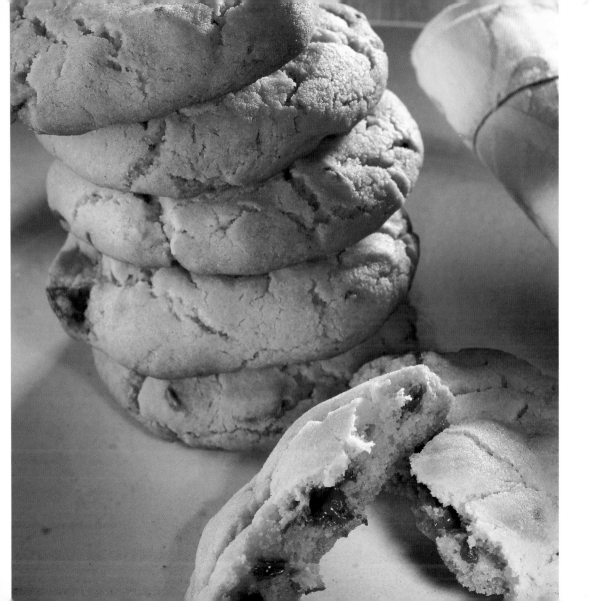

Counting Calories: Breads & Baked Products

	Typical portion	Typical portion size	Calories per portion	Calories per 100 g/ml	Fat per 100 g/ml	Health rating (1–10)
Jammie creams	1	19 g/⅔ oz	85	**448**	16.7	2
Lemon puffs	1	13 g/½ oz	69	**533**	31.2	2
Lemon thins	1	10 g/¼ oz	47	**468**	17.3	2
Lincoln biscuits	1	8 g/¼ oz	40	**479**	20.6	2
Macaroons, coconut	1	33 g/1⅙ oz	146	**441**	18.6	3
Macaroons, French	1	60 g/2 oz	225	**375**	18.3	3
Malted milk biscuits	1	8 g/¼ oz	39	**490**	22.0	2
Malted milk biscuits, chocolate	1	11 g/¼ oz	56	**509**	25.0	2
Nice biscuits	1	8 g/¼ oz	34	**485**	20.8	2
Oat and raisin cookies	1	12 g/³⁄₇ oz	50	**414**	8.8	4
Oat-based biscuits	1	16 g/⁴⁄₇ oz	75	**468**	21.4	3
Oatcakes	1	16 g/⁴⁄₇ oz	71	**441**	16.9	6
Rice cakes, low fat	1	9 g/¼ oz	34	**374**	2.2	4
Rich tea biscuits	1	10 g/¼ oz	39	**430**	10.6	2
Rich tea biscuits, milk chocolate	1	13 g/½ oz	65	**497**	23.0	2
Rich tea finger	1	5 g/⅙ oz	23	**451**	14.4	2
Sandwich biscuits, cream filled	1	14/½ oz	72	**516**	25.8	2
Semi-sweet biscuits	1	10 g/¼ oz	43	**427**	13.3	2
Short sweet biscuits	1	10 g/¼ oz	45	**454**	21.8	2
Shortbread fingers	1	20 g/¾ oz	100	**498**	26.1	2
Shortbread, caramel and chocolate	1	55 g/2 oz	245	**446**	27.7	2
Shortcake	1	10 g/¼ oz	56	**506**	25.1	3

	Typical portion	Typical portion size	Calories per portion	Calories per 100 g/ml	Fat per 100 g/ml	Health rating (1–10)
Viennese-style biscuits	1	32 g/1⅛ oz	167	**523**	31.8	2
Wafer biscuits	1	8 g/¼ oz	43	**537**	30.1	3
Wafers, filled, chocolate, full coated	1	20 g/¾ oz	102	**513**	29.7	2
Water biscuits	1	8 g/¼ oz	35	**440**	12.5	3
Cakes						
Almond slices	1	35 g/1¼ oz	141	**403**	13.4	3
Angel cake	1 slice	41 g/1½ oz	171	**417**	19.8	3
Bakewell slices	1	35 g/1¼ oz	153	**436**	20.4	3
Bakewell, cherry (individual)	1	44 g/1⅝ oz	185	**420**	17.7	3
Banana loaf	1 slice	40 g/1½ oz	151	**377**	19.5	4
Banana loaf, date and walnut	1 slice	28 g/1 oz	78	**280**	4.9	4
Battenburg cake	1 slice	35 g/1¼ oz	119	**339**	7.0	3
Carrot cake	1 slice	40 g/1½ oz	144	**359**	14.3	4
Carrot and orange cake	1 slice	47 g/1⅔ oz	165	**350**	15.7	4
Christmas cake	1 slice	60 g/2 oz	216	**360**	9.2	4
Coconut cake	1 slice	70 g/2½ oz	304	**434**	23.8	3
Cupcakes, chocolate	1	38 g/1⅓ oz	170	**448**	24.0	2
Cupcakes, lemon	1	38 g/1⅓ oz	116	**305**	2.1	2
Cupcakes, pink	1	38 g/1⅓ oz	155	**410**	8.5	2
Custard slice	1	108 g/3⅘ oz	320	**296**	15.2	2
Date and walnut loaf	1 slice	40 g/1½ oz	148	**371**	20.4	4
Double chocolate ganache cake	1 slice	61 g/2⅐ oz	281	**460**	27.6	2

Counting Calories: Breads & Baked Products

	Typical portion	Typical portion size	Calories per portion	Calories per 100 g/ml	Fat per 100 g/ml	Health rating (1–10)
Dundee cake	1 slice	75 g/3 oz	254	**339**	11.0	4
Eclairs, chocolate, with fresh cream	1	59 g/2 oz	210	**356**	26.7	2
Fairy cake	1	16 g/⅗ oz	70	**436**	21.9	2
Fondant fancy	1	27 g/1 oz	95	**353**	9.0	2
Fruit cake, plain	1 slice	90 g/3¼ oz	319	**354**	12.9	4
Fruit cake, rich	1 slice	90 g/3¼ oz	293	**326**	10.0	4
Fruit cake, rich, iced	1 slice	70 g/2½ oz	249	**356**	11.4	4
Fruit cake, wholemeal	1 slice	65 g/2½ oz	238	**366**	16.2	3
Fudge cake, chocolate	1 slice	60 g/2 oz	230	**382**	16.2	2
Gateau, Black Forest	1 slice	56 g/2 oz	126	**225**	11.0	5
Gateau, chocolate	1 slice	100 g/3½ oz	176	**176**	10.0	2
Gateau, double chocolate	1 slice	85 g/3 oz	281	**331**	16.5	2
Gateau, strawberry	1 slice	85 g/3 oz	200	**235**	13.6	2
Gingerbread	1 piece	50 g/2 oz	190	**379**	12.6	4
Jaffa cakes	1	22 g/⅞ oz	83	**377**	8.1	2
Jamaica ginger cake	1 slice	60 g/2 oz	216	**360**	10.8	3
Madeira cake	1 slice	65 g/2½ oz	245	**377**	15.1	3
Muffins, American style, choc. chip	1	72 g/2½ oz	284	**395**	20.0	2
Rock cake	1 small	40 g/1½ oz	158	**396**	16.4	3
Sponge cake	1 slice	53 g/2 oz	243	**459**	26.3	2
Sponge cake, made without fat	1 slice	53 g/2 oz	156	**294**	6.1	2
Sponge cake, jam filled	1 slice	65 g/2½ oz	196	**302**	4.9	2

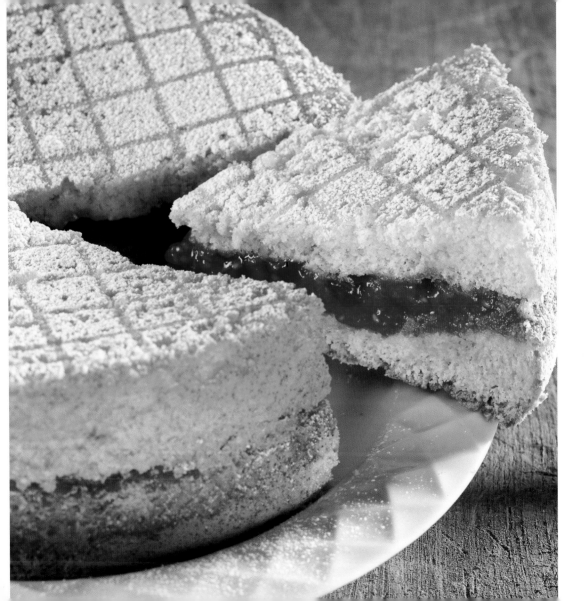

	Typical portion	Typical portion size	Calories per portion	Calories per 100 g/ml	Fat per 100 g/ml	Health rating (1–10)
Sponge cake, with dairy cream and jam	1 slice	60 g/2 oz	170	**284**	10.0	2
Sponge roll, chocolate	1 piece	66 g/2½ oz	251	**380**	18.4	2
Swiss roll, chocolate	1 piece	50 g/2 oz	189	**379**	19.3	2
Swiss roll, chocolate, mini	1	22 g/⅞ oz	87	**396**	14.8	2
Victoria sponge, chocolate	1 slice	61 g/2½ oz	201	**330**	16.0	2
Victoria sponge, fresh cream	1 slice	50 g/2 oz	168	**337**	17.4	2
Walnut and coffee cake	1 slice	65 g/2½ oz	253	**390**	20.0	3
Pastry Dough						
Flaky pastry, raw	n/a	n/a	n/a	**427**	31.1	3
Flaky pastry, cooked	n/a	n/a	n/a	**564**	41.0	3
Puff pastry, frozen	n/a	n/a	n/a	**400**	25.6	3
Shortcrust pastry, raw	n/a	n/a	n/a	**451**	28.1	3
Shortcrust pastry, cooked	n/a	n/a	n/a	**524**	32.6	3
Wholemeal pastry, raw	n/a	n/a	n/a	**433**	28.7	5
Wholemeal pastry, cooked	n/a	n/a	n/a	**501**	33.2	5
Pizza base, deep pan	1	220 g/7¾ oz	684	**311**	5.0	3
Pizza base, light and crispy	1	150 g/5 oz	437	**291**	3.0	3
Buns and Pastries						
Baklava	1 bag	50 g/2 oz	194	**393**	21.0	2
Bath bun	1	80 g/3 oz	262	**327**	11.1	3
Chelsea bun	1	78 g/3 oz	288	**368**	14.2	2
Cream horn	1	57 g/2 oz	244	**428**	27.8	3

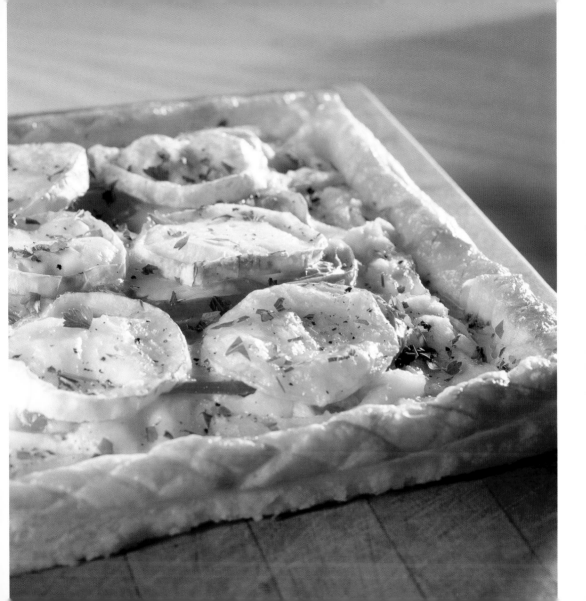

Counting Calories: Breads & Baked Products

	Typical portion	Typical portion size	Calories per portion	Calories per 100 g/ml	Fat per 100 g/ml	Health rating (1–10)
Currant bun	1	60 g/2 oz	168	**280**	5.6	1
Custard tart, individual	1	67 g/2½ oz	186	**277**	14.5	2
Danish pastry	1	49 g/1¾ oz	287	**428**	26.0	2
Danish pastry, apple	1	67 g/2½ oz	248	**368**	21.6	2
Danish pastry, apple and cinnamon	1	67 g/2½ oz	193	**288**	1.9	2
Danish pastry, apple and sultana	1	67 g/2½ oz	273	**407**	22.8	2
Danish pastry, cherry and custard	1	67 g/2½ oz	174	**260**	14.0	2
Danish pastry, pecan	1	67 g/2½ oz	287	**428**	26.0	2
Danish pastry, fruit-filled	1	67 g/2½ oz	239	**356**	16.9	2
Doughnuts, jam	1	80 g/3 oz	268	**336**	14.5	1
Doughnuts, ring, plain	1	60 g/2 oz	238	**397**	21.7	1
Doughnuts, apple and fresh cream	1	79 g/3 oz	216	**273**	14.4	1
Doughnuts, chocolate	1	60 g/2 oz	214	**356**	16.6	1
Doughnuts, jam and cream	1	90 g/3¼ oz	288	**320**	15.7	1
Doughnuts, apple and custard	1	90 g/3¼ oz	254	**282**	13.9	1
Doughnut fingers, with cream	1	90 g/3¼ oz	93	**349**	20.1	1
Doughnuts, ring, iced	1	70 g/2½ oz	268	**383**	17.5	1
Doughnuts (yum yums)	1	37 g/1⅓ oz	155	**420**	23.9	1
Eccles cakes	1	45 g/1⅗ oz	171	**387**	17.8	3
Eclairs, frozen	1	35 g/1¼ oz	139	**396**	30.6	2
Greek pastries	1	35 g/1¼ oz	113	**322**	17.0	2
Hot cross bun	1	80 g/3 oz	223	**279**	6.7	3

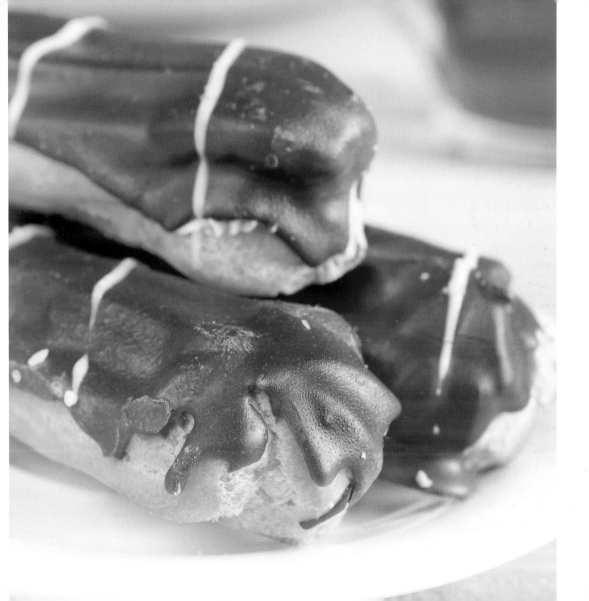

Counting Calories: Breads & Baked Products

	Typical portion	Typical portion size	Calories per portion	Calories per 100 g/ml	Fat per 100 g/ml	Health rating (1–10)
Hot cross bun, wholemeal	1	80 g/3 oz	210	**262**	6.0	5
Iced bun	1	80 g/3 oz	240	**300**	3.7	2
Jam tarts	1	35 g/1¼ oz	134	**383**	14.7	2
Mince pies, individual	1	50 g/2 oz	218	**435**	21.3	3
Pain au chocolat	1	53 g/2 oz	230	**435**	23.9	1
Pain au raisin	1	53 g/2 oz	203	**383**	19.0	2
Scotch pancakes (drop scones)	1	50 g/2 oz	135	**270**	9.6	3
Teacakes, toasted	1	60 g/2 oz	198	**329**	8.3	3
Cereal Bars						
Cereal bar, chewy	1	35 g/1¼ oz	146	**419**	16.4	3
Cereal bar, crunchy	1	35 g/1¼ oz	164	**468**	22.2	3
Flapjacks, all butter	1	35 g/1¼ oz	156	**446**	22.8	3
Flapjacks, caramel bake	½	45 g/1⅜ oz	188	**417**	14.5	3
Flapjacks, cherry and coconut	½	45 g/1⅜ oz	200	**445**	21.0	4
Flapjacks, chocolate chip	½	45 g/1⅜ oz	188	**417**	15.0	3
Flapjacks, cranberry, apple and raisin	½	45 g/1⅜ oz	146	**325**	5.6	4
Flapjacks, raspberry	½	45 g/1⅜ oz	189	**420**	18.0	4
Raw fruit and nut bar	1	35 g/1¼ oz	143	**410**	23.0	7
Seed bar	1	50 g/2 oz	277	**555**	40.6	5
Savoury Products						
Blinis, cocktail	1	12 g/⅜ oz	23	**190**	2.3	3
Blinis with sausage	1	16 g/½ oz	30	**190**	2.3	2

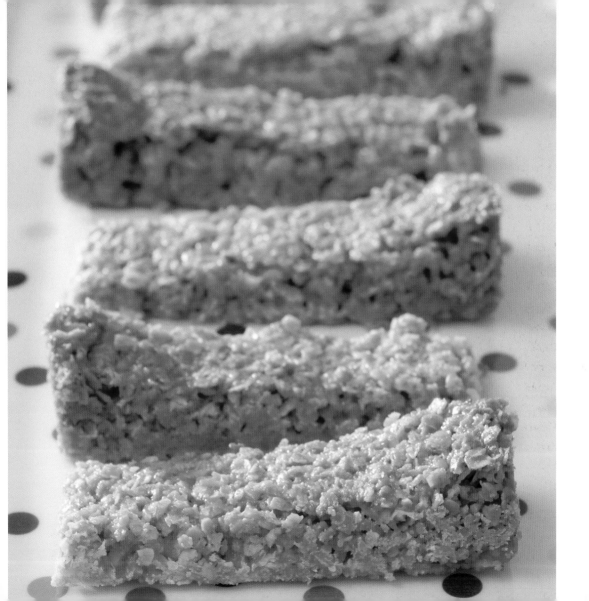

Counting Calories: Breads & Baked Products

	Typical portion	Typical portion size	Calories per portion	Calories per 100 g/ml	Fat per 100 g/ml	Health rating (1–10)
Blinis with smoked salmon	1	25 g/1 oz	60	**240**	13.0	3
Bruschetta with ploughman's relish	1 pack	90 g/3¼ oz	261	**290**	17.2	4
Bruschetta with red pepper and onion	1 pack	90 g/3¼ oz	267	**296**	19.0	4
Bruschetta with soft cheese and cranberry	1 pack	90 g/3¼ oz	190	**211**	9.0	4
Calzone, bolognese, healthy range	1	88 g/3⅛ oz	178	**202**	3.4	4
Calzone, cheese and tomato, healthy range	1	88 g/3⅛ oz	191	**217**	4.3	4
Calzone, ham and Gruyère	1	280 g/10 oz	661	**236**	8.0	4
Canapés, Aegean tomato	1	15 g/½ oz	45	**300**	14.7	4
Canapés, caponata	1	15 g/½ oz	38	**249**	15.7	4
Canapés, salmon and dill	1	15 g/½ oz	47	**315**	16.1	4
Canapés, smoked salmon	1	15 g/½ oz	32	**210**	15.2	4
Cheese and onion rolls, pastry	1	140 g/5 oz	458	**327**	20.0	2
Croutons	1 tbsp	20 g/¾ oz	106	**530**	32.8	2
Doughballs, cheese and garlic	1	15 g/½ oz	51	**341**	18.5	2
Doughballs, garlic	1	15 g/½ oz	52	**347**	16.4	2
Doughballs, garlic and herb	1	15 g/½ oz	52	**343**	17.2	2
Dumplings	1	50 g/2 oz	192	**384**	17.6	2
Dumplings, dry mix	1 pack	150 g/5 oz	443	**295**	12.2	2
Dumplings, pork, garlic and chive	1	50 g/2 oz	94	**187**	7.0	2
Dumplings, prawn, Cantonese	1	10 g/¼ oz	24	**241**	13.4	2
Gnocchi	½ pack	50 g/2 oz	74	**148**	0.2	2
Pancakes, savoury, made with whole milk	1	77 g/3 oz	210	**273**	17.5	4

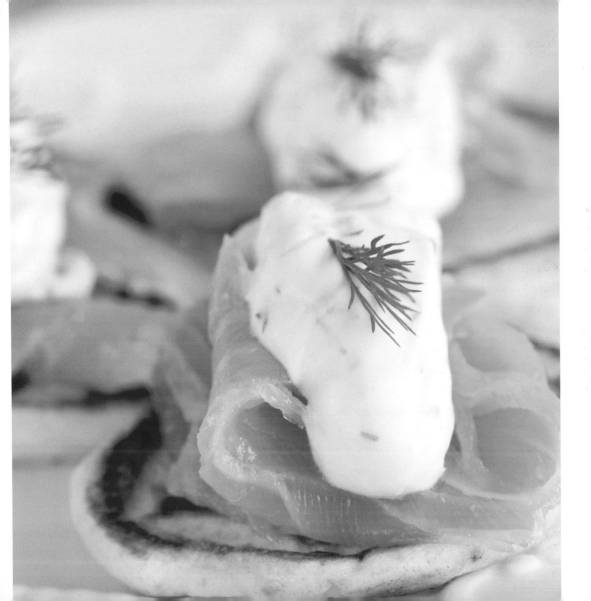

	Typical portion	Typical portion size	Calories per portion	Calories per 100 g/ml	Fat per 100 g/ml	Health rating (1–10)
Vol-au-vents, garlic mushroom	1	19 g/⅔ oz	66	**347**	27.0	3
Vol-au-vents, mushroom	1	19 g/⅔ oz	67	**350**	22.1	3
Vol-au-vents, seafood	1	19 g/⅔ oz	67	**354**	24.8	3
Yorkshire pudding	1 bag	25 g/1 oz	53	**210**	10.1	3

Savoury Pies – *see* page 227 for sweet pies

Beef, minced	⅓	100 g/3½ oz	255	**255**	15.6	4
Beef and vegetable	⅓	100 g/3½ oz	256	**256**	116.9	3
Cheese and onion	⅓	100 g/3½ oz	258	**258**	12.2	4
Chicken, leek and ham	⅓	100 g/3½ oz	270	**270**	14.7	3
Chicken, individual, chilled/frozen, baked	1	170 g/6 oz	489	**288**	17.7	3
Cottage	⅓	100 g/3½ oz	115	**115**	5.6	5
Cumberland	⅓	100 g/3½ oz	160	**160**	10.4	5
Fish pie, cod and smoked haddock	½	200 g/7 oz	160	**80**	2.4	6
Fisherman's	1	248 g/8¾ oz	335	**135**	6.4	6
Admiral's, frozen	½ pack	180 g/6⅓ oz	189	**105**	4.9	4
Fish and prawn	⅓	10 g/¼ oz	101	**101**	3.6	6
Game	⅙	125 g/4 oz	351	**381**	22.5	4
Lamb and mint	⅓	100 g/3½ oz	275	**275**	17.4	4
Meat and potato	⅓	100 g/3½ oz	288	**288**	18.4	3
Pasty, cheese and onion	1	200 g/7 oz	546	**546**	21.1	3
Pasty, chicken and vegetable	1	255 g/9 oz	671	**263**	13.6	4
Pasty, Cornish, traditional	1	200 g/7 oz	592	**296**	18.4	3

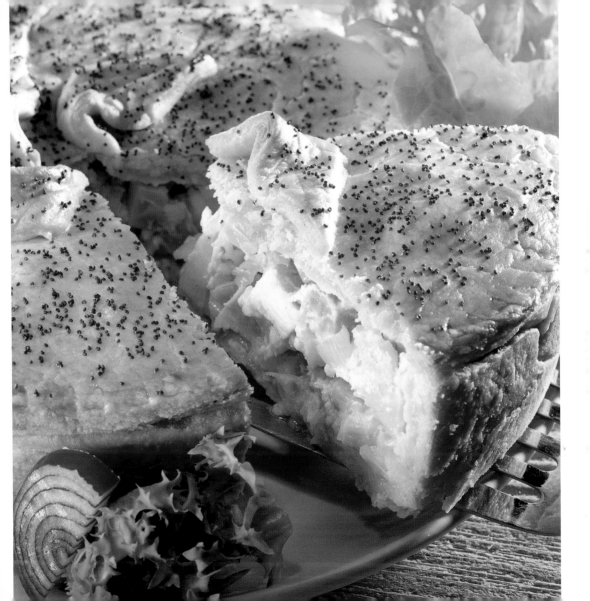

Counting Calories: Breads & Baked Products

	Typical portion	Typical portion size	Calories per portion	Calories per 100 g/ml	Fat per 100 g/ml	Health rating (1–10)
Pasty, vegetable	1	200 g/7 oz	454	**227**	11.3	3
Pork pie, individual	1	110 g/4 oz	399	**363**	25.7	2
Pork and egg	⅓	100 g/3½ oz	351	**351**	25.9	2
Roast chicken and vegetable	⅓	100 g/3½ oz	200	**200**	12.5	4
Shepherd's	⅓	100 g/3½ oz	126	**126**	6.0	6
Steak and kidney, single crust, home-made	⅙	125 g/4 oz	327	**261**	15.1	4
Steak and kidney/beef, chilled/frozen, baked	1	150 g/6 oz	465	**310**	19.4	3
Steak, in rich gravy	⅓	100 g/3½ oz	264	**264**	15.2	4
Steak and kidney	⅓	100 g/3½ oz	282	**282**	15.7	4
Steak and kidney, tinned	⅓	100 g/3½ oz	163	**163**	8.8	3
Steak and mushroom	⅓	100 g/3½ oz	286	**286**	16.4	4
Vegetable, individual	1	120 g/4 oz	191	**159**	8.4	3
Vegetable	⅓	100 g/3½ oz	151	**151**	7.6	4

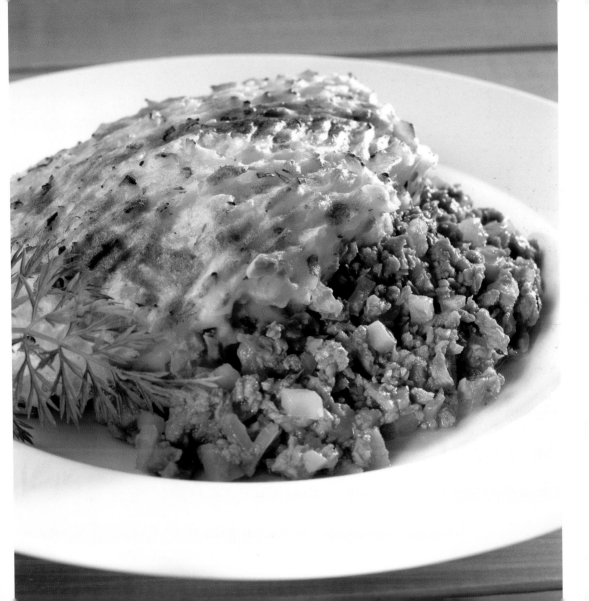

Alcohol & Beverages

	Typical portion	Typical portion size	Calories per portion	Calories per 100 g/ml	Fat per 100 g/ml	Health rating (1–10)
Coffee						
Café latte, fast food, regular size	1	337 ml/11⅔ fl oz	135	**41**	1.0	3
Café latte, mocha, with skimmed milk	1 mug	227 ml/8 fl oz	208	**83**	0.7	4
Café latte, mocha, with semi-skimmed milk	1 mug	227 ml/8 fl oz	218	**87**	1.0	4
Café latte, with skimmed milk, retail	1 mug	227 ml/8 fl oz	85	**34**	0.3	4
Café latte, with semi-skimmed milk, retail	1 mug	227 ml/8 fl oz	115	**46**	1.7	4
Cappuccino, fast food, regular size	1	231 ml/8½ fl oz	90	**39**	1.0	3
Cappuccino, retail	1 mug	227 ml/8 fl oz	98	**39**	1.0	3
Fast food, with milk, regular size	1	313 ml/1 fl oz	25	**8**	0.1	3
Frappuccino, caramel, grande	1 cup	473 ml/16 fl oz	294	**62**	0.8	2
Frappuccino, coffee, grande	1 cup	473 ml/16 fl oz	261	**55**	2.0	3
Frappuccino, espresso, grande	1 cup	473 ml/16 fl oz	209	**44**	0.6	4
Frappuccino, mocha, light, grande	1 cup	473 ml/16 fl oz	144	**30**	0.3	4
Frappuccino, vanilla with whipped cream, grande	1 cup	473 ml/16 fl oz	460	**97**	3.6	2
Infusion, with water	1 cup	220 ml/8 fl oz	4.4	**2**	0.0	2
Infusion, with whole milk	1 cup	220 ml/8 fl oz	15.4	**7**	0.4	3
Instant, black	1 mug	227 ml/8 fl oz	0	**0**	0.0	1
Instant, with semi-skimmed milk	1 mug	227 ml/8 fl oz	13	**7**	0.2	1
Instant, with whole milk	1 mug	227 ml/8 fl oz	13	**7**	0.4	3

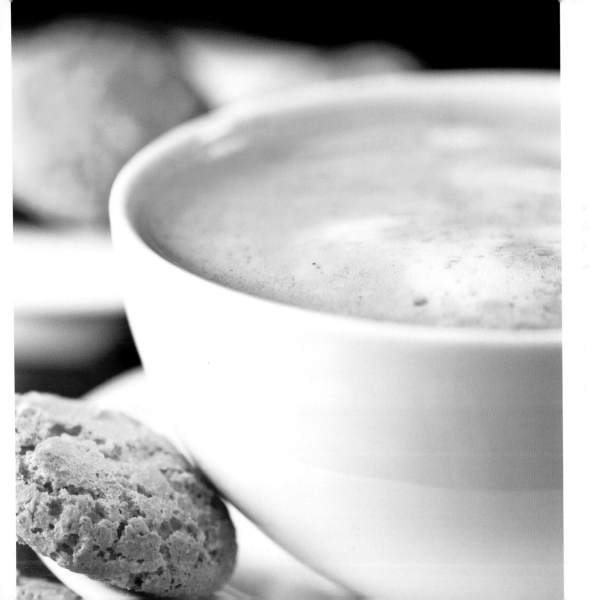

	Typical portion	Typical portion size	Calories per portion	Calories per 100 g/ml	Fat per 100 g/ml	Health rating (1–10)
Instant, with cream	1 mug	227 ml/8 fl oz	35	**14**	1.2	2
Tea						
Black, no milk	1 mug	227 ml/8 fl oz	3	**1**	0.0	2
Black, decaf, no milk	1 mug	227 ml/8 fl oz	3	**1**	0.0	3
Black, with skimmed milk	1 mug	227 ml/8 fl oz	15	**6**	0.2	3
Black, with semi-skimmed milk	1 mug	227 ml/8 fl oz	18	**7**	0.2	3
Black, with whole milk	1 mug	227 ml/8 fl oz	27	**11**	0.2	3
Black, fast food, with milk	1	333 ml/11⅝ fl oz	10	**3**	0.1	4
Camomile	1 mug	227 ml/8 fl oz	5	**2**	0.0	3
Fruit	1 mug	227 ml/8 fl oz	13	**5**	0.0	3
Green	1 mug	227 ml/8 fl oz	0	**0**	0.0	3
Green and lemon, iced	1 mug	250 ml/8¾ fl oz	75	**30**	0.1	5
Hot Chocolate and Malt						
Cocoa powder	1 dssp	16 g/⅝ oz	50	**312**	21.7	3
Drinking chocolate powder	1 dssp	16 g/⅝ oz	64	**402**	2.4	3
Drink. choc. powder, made up with skim. milk	1 mug	227 ml/8 fl oz	100	**44**	0.5	5
Drink. choc. powder, made up with s.-skim. milk	1 mug	227 ml/8 fl oz	129	**57**	1.9	5
Drink. choc. powder, made up with whole milk	1 mug	227 ml/8 fl oz	173	**76**	4.2	4
Hot chocolate, fast food	1	330 ml/11 fl oz	164	**50**	1.1	3
Malted milk drink, light, made up with skim. milk	1 mug	227 ml/8 fl oz	159	**70**	0.5	5
Malted milk drink, light, made up with s.-skim. milk	1 mug	227 ml/8 fl oz	184	**81**	1.9	5
Malted milk drink, light, made up with whole milk	1 mug	227 ml/8 fl oz	225	**99**	3.9	4

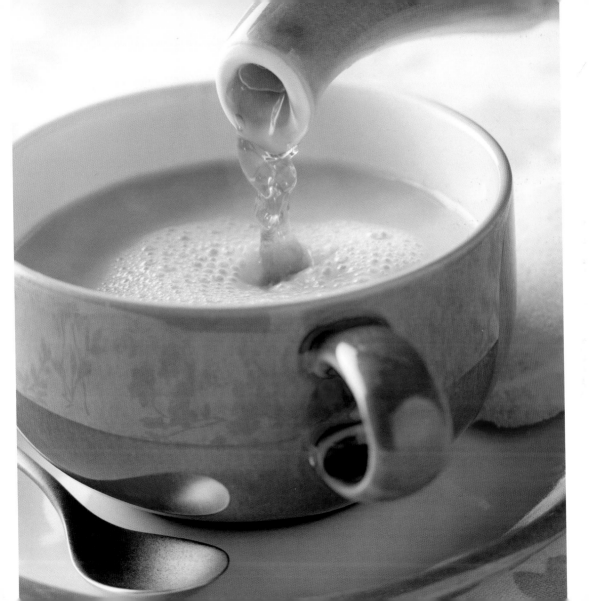

	Typical portion	Typical portion size	Calories per portion	Calories per 100 g/ml	Fat per 100 g/ml	Health rating (1–10)
Malted milk powder, low fat	2 tbsp	32 g/1⅛ oz	116	**364**	3.8	3
Instant drinks powder, chocolate, low calorie	2 tbsp	32 g/1⅛ oz	115	**359**	11.1	3
Instant drinks powder, malted	2 tbsp	32 g/1⅛ oz	133	**416**	9.5	3

Milk Shakes – see Eggs, Dairy & Fats, page 42

Fizzy Soft Drinks

	Typical portion	Typical portion size	Calories per portion	Calories per 100 g/ml	Fat per 100 g/ml	Health rating (1–10)
Bitter lemon	1 glass	150 ml/¼ pint	51	**34**	0.0	1
Bitter lemon, low calorie	1 glass	150 ml/¼ pint	5	**3**	0.1	2
Cola	1 can	330 ml/11⅔ fl oz	135	**41**	0.0	1
Cola, diet and caffeine free	1 can	330 ml/11⅔ fl oz	1	**0**	0.0	3
Cream soda, American, with vanilla	1 glass	250 ml/8¾ fl oz	60	**24**	0.0	1
Cream soda, traditional	1 glass	250 ml/8¾ fl oz	105	**42**	0.0	1
Cream soda, diet	1 glass	250 ml/8¾ fl oz	3	**1**	0.0	2
Dandelion and burdock	1 can	330 ml/11⅔ fl oz	98	**29**	0.0	2
Dandelion and burdock, diet	1 can	330 ml/11⅔ fl oz	4	**1**	0.0	2
Energy drink (e.g. Lucozade)	1 bottle	500 ml/18 fl oz	350	**70**	0.0	1
Fruit juice drink (e.g. Fanta)	1 can	330 ml/11⅔ fl oz	129	**39**	0.0	2
Ginger beer	1 can	330 ml/11⅔ fl oz	115	**35**	0.0	2
Ginger beer, light	1 can	330 ml/11⅔ fl oz	3	**1**	0.0	1
Lemonade	1 glass	250 ml/8¾ fl oz	52	**21**	0.1	1
Lemonade, low calorie/diet	1 glass	250 ml/8¾ fl oz	7.3	**3**	0.0	2
Ginger ale, American	1 glass	150 ml/¼ pint	100	**67**	0.0	1
Ginger ale, American, low calorie	1 glass	150 ml/¼ pint	1	**1**	0.0	1

	Typical portion	Typical portion size	Calories per portion	Calories per 100 g/ml	Fat per 100 g/ml	Health rating (1–10)
Ginger ale, dry	1 glass	150 ml/¼ pint	37	**15**	0.0	1
Tonic water, Indian	1 glass	150 ml/¼ pint	33	**22**	0.0	1
Tonic water, Indian, slimline	1 glass	150 ml/¼ pint	3	**2**	0.0	1
Squash and Cordials						
Blackcurrant juice drink, concentrated	1 dssp	10 ml/⅓ fl oz	23	**228**	0.0	3
Elderflower juice drink, concentrated	1 dssp	10 ml/⅓ fl oz	11	**110**	0.0	1
Fruit drink/squash, concentrated	1 dssp	10 ml/⅓ fl oz	10	**93**	0.0	3
Fruit drink, low calorie, diluted	1 glass	250 ml/8¾ fl oz	8	**3**	0.0	3
Fruit juice drink, ready to drink	1 glass	250 ml/8¾ fl oz	93	**37**	0.0	3
Fruit juice drink, low calorie, ready to drink	1 glass	250 ml/8¾ fl oz	25	**10**	0.0	3
Lemonade, still, fresh	1 glass	250 ml/8¾ fl oz	100	**40**	0.2	5
Lime juice cordial, concentrated	1 dssp	10 ml/⅓ fl oz	13	**112**	0.0	3
Juices						
Apple juice, concentrate	1 tbsp	15 ml/½ fl oz	45	**302**	0.1	5
Apple juice, unsweetened	1 glass	150 ml/¼ pint	57	**38**	0.1	6
Carrot juice	1 glass	150 ml/¼ pint	35	**23**	0.0	6
Cranberry juice	1 glass	150 ml/¼ pint	92	**61**	0.1	6
Fruit smoothie, average	1 glass	250 ml/8¾ fl oz	143	**58**	0.1	6
Grape juice, unsweetened	1 glass	150 ml/¼ pint	69	**46**	0.1	5
Grapefruit juice, unsweetened	1 glass	150 ml/¼ pint	50	**33**	0.1	5
Lemon juice, fresh	1 dssp	10 ml/⅓ fl oz	1	**7**	0.0	4
Lime juice	1 dssp	10 ml/⅓ fl oz	1	**9**	0.1	4

Counting Calories: Alcohol & Beverages

	Typical portion	Typical portion size	Calories per portion	Calories per 100 g/ml	Fat per 100 g/ml	Health rating (1–10)
Orange juice, unsweetened	1 glass	150 ml/¼ pint	54	**36**	0.1	5
Orange juice, concentrate, unsweetened	1 glass	150 ml/¼ pint	278	**185**	0.5	5
Pineapple juice, unsweetened	1 glass	150 ml/¼ pint	62	**41**	0.1	5
Prune juice	1 glass	150 ml/¼ pint	92	**61**	0.1	6
Tomato juice	1 glass	150 ml/¼ pint	21	**14**	0.0	6
Beers						
Ale, strong, bottled	1 bottle	330 ml/11⅔ fl oz	148	**45**	0.0	3
Ale, brown, bottled	1 bottle	330 ml/11⅔ fl oz	99	**30**	0.0	3
Ale, pale, bottled	1 bottle	330 ml/11⅔ fl oz	92	**28**	0.0	3
Ale, strong (barley wine)	⅓ pint	189 ml/6⅔ fl oz	125	**66**	0.0	3
Beer, low carb	1 glass	250 ml/8¾ fl oz	77	**31**	0.0	3
Beer, mild, draught	1 pint	568 ml/1 pint	136	**24**	0.0	3
Beer, non-alcoholic	1 bottle	330 ml/11 fl oz	79	**24**	0.0	3
Bitter, canned	1 can	440 ml/15 fl oz	141	**32**	0.0	2
Bitter, draught	1 pint	568 ml/1 pint	182	**32**	0.0	3
Bitter, low alcohol	1 pint	568 ml/1 pint	74	**13**	0.0	2
Lager	1 pint	568 ml/1 pint	233	**41**	0.0	1
Lager, non-alcoholic	1 bottle	275 ml/9⅔ fl oz	55	**20**	0.0	2
Lager, low alcohol	1 can	440 ml/¾ pint	44	**10**	0.0	1
Lager, low carb	1 bottle	275 ml/9⅔ fl oz	88	**32**	0.0	1
Lager, premium	1 can	440 ml/¾ pint	260	**59**	0.0	1
Shandy	1 pint	568 ml/1 pint	136	**24**	0.0	1

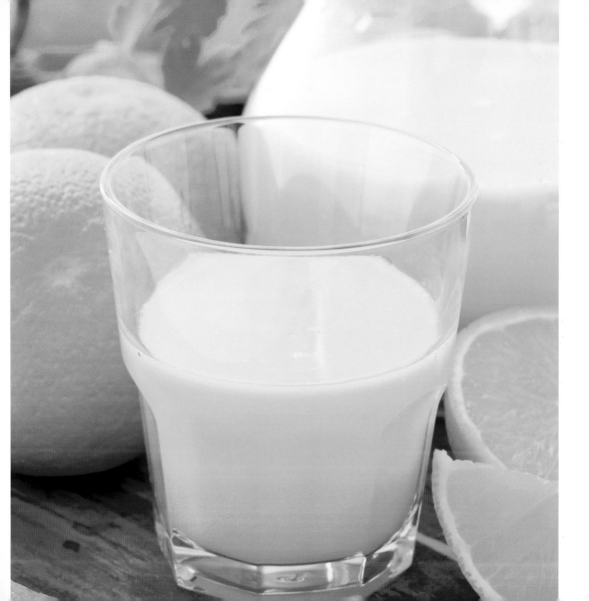

Counting Calories: Alcohol & Beverages

	Typical portion	Typical portion size	Calories per portion	Calories per 100 g/ml	Fat per 100 g/ml	Health rating (1–10)
Stout	1 pint	568 ml/1 pint	170	**30**	0.0	3
Stout, Irish, dry, draught	1 pint	568 ml/1 pint	210	**37**	0.0	3
Stout, Irish, dry, bottled	1 bottle	500 ml/18 fl oz	215	**43**	0.0	3
Ciders						
Cider, dry	1 pint	568 ml/1 pint	204	**36**	0.0	2
Cider, low alcohol	1 pint	568 ml/1 pint	97	**17**	0.0	2
Cider, pear	½ pint	284 ml/½ pint	122	**43**	0.0	2
Cider, sweet	1 pint	568 ml/1 pint	239	**42**	0.0	1
Cider, vintage	1 pint	568 ml/1 pint	573	**101**	0.0	2
Scrumpy	1 pint	568 ml/1 pint	261	**46**	0.0	1
Wines						
Champagne	1 glass	120 ml/4 fl oz	107	**89**	0.0	2
Red wine	1 glass	120 ml/4 fl oz	82	**68**	0.0	4
Rosé wine, medium	1 glass	120 ml/4 fl oz	85	**71**	0.0	4
White wine, dry	1 glass	120 ml/4 fl oz	79	**66**	0.0	3
White wine, medium	1 glass	120 ml/4 fl oz	89	**74**	0.0	3
White wine, sparkling	1 glass	120 ml/4 fl oz	89	**74**	0.0	3
White wine, sweet	1 glass	120 ml/4 fl oz	113	**94**	0.0	3
Fortified Wine						
Port	1 measure	50 ml/2 fl oz	79	**157**	0.0	3
Sherry, dry	1 measure	50 ml/2 fl oz	58	**116**	0.0	2
Sherry, medium	1 measure	50 ml/2 fl oz	58	**116**	0.0	2

	Typical portion	Typical portion size	Calories per portion	Calories per 100 g/ml	Fat per 100 g/ml	Health rating (1–10)
Sherry, sweet	1 measure	50 ml/2 fl oz	68	**136**	0.0	2
Vermouth, dry	1 measure	50 ml/2 fl oz	55	**109**	0.0	1
Vermouth, sweet	1 measure	50 ml/2 fl oz	76	**151**	0.0	1
Liqueurs						
Advocaat	1 measure	35 ml/1¼ fl oz	91	**260**	6.3	1
Amaretto	1 measure	35 ml/1¼ fl oz	135	**388**	0.0	1
Coffee	1 measure	35 ml/1¼ fl oz	105	**300**	0.0	1
Cream	1 measure	35 ml/1¼ fl oz	114	**325**	16.1	1
Cream, Irish	1 measure	35 ml/1¼ fl oz	114	**327**	13.0	1
Curaçao	1 measure	35 ml/1¼ fl oz	109	**311**	0.0	1
Curaçao, triple sec (e.g. Cointreau)	1 measure	35 ml/1¼ fl oz	75	**215**	0.0	1
Generic, high strength	1 measure	35 ml/1¼ fl oz	110	**314**	0.0	1
Generic, medium strength	1 measure	35 ml/1¼ fl oz	92	**262**	0.0	1
Grand Marnier	1 measure	35 ml/1¼ fl oz	94	**268**	0.0	1
Pastis (e.g. Pernod)	1 measure	35 ml/1¼ fl oz	46	**130**	0.0	1
Peach	1 measure	35 ml/1¼ fl oz	91	**260**	0.0	1
Whiskey/bourbon (e.g. Southern Comfort)	1 measure	35 ml/1¼ fl oz	72	**207**	0.0	1
Whisky (e.g. Drambuie)	1 measure	35 ml/1¼ fl oz	95	**272**	0.0	1
Spirits						
Absinthe	1 measure	35 ml/1¼ fl oz	127	**363**	0.0	1
Brandy, 40% volume	1 measure	35 ml/1¼ fl oz	78	**222**	0.0	1
Fruit cup (e.g. Pimm's No. 1 Cup)	1 measure	35 ml/1¼ fl oz	56	**160**	0.0	1

Counting Calories: Alcohol & Beverages

	Typical portion	Typical portion size	Calories per portion	Calories per 100 g/ml	Fat per 100 g/ml	Health rating (1–10)
Generic (including whisky and gin), 40% vol.	1 measure	35 ml/1¼ fl oz	78	**222**	0.0	1
Gin and tonic, premixed, can	1 can	250 ml/8¾ fl oz	213	**85**	0.0	1
Kirsch	1 measure	35 ml/1¼ fl oz	93	**267**	0.0	1
Rum, white	1 measure	35 ml/1¼ fl oz	72	**207**	0.0	1
Sake (rice wine)	1 measure	35 ml/1¼ fl oz	47	**134**	0.0	1
Sambuca	1 measure	35 ml/1¼ fl oz	122	**348**	0.0	1
Tequila	1 measure	35 ml/1¼ fl oz	78	**224**	0.0	1
Vodka	1 measure	35 ml/1¼ fl oz	78	**222**	0.0	1
Whiskey/bourbon, 86% proof	1 measure	35 ml/1¼ fl oz	88	**250**	0.0	1

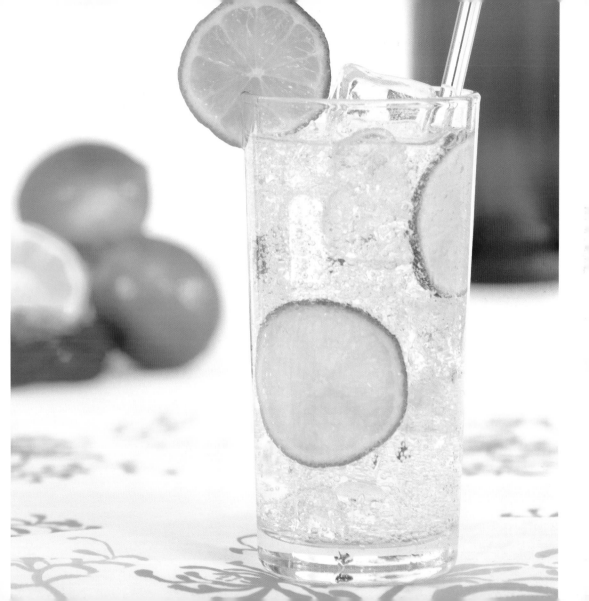

Snacks, Confectionery & Desserts

	Typical portion	Typical portion size	Calories per portion	Calories per 100 g/ml	Fat per 100 g/ml	Health rating (1–10)
Sandwiches						
Bacon/egg; bacon/tomato; sausage/egg (triple)	1 pack	256 g/9 oz	778	**304**	20.8	4
Bacon, lettuce and tomato	1 pack	181 g/6⅜ oz	425	**235**	12.4	5
Beef and horseradish	1 pack	187 g/6⅗ oz	389	**208**	7.3	5
Breakfast, big, with ketchup	1 pack	206 g/7¼ oz	546	**265**	13.4	3
Cheese and pickle	1 pack	171 g/6 oz	588	**344**	15.8	4
Chicken fajita wrap	1 pack	185 g/6½ oz	263	**142**	2.2	4
Chicken salad	1 pack	208 g/7⅓ oz	406	**195**	9.5	5
Chicken salad, healthy range	1 pack	195 g/7 oz	257	**132**	2.5	5
Chicken; ham; prawn (triple)	1 pack	247 g/8⁵⁄₇ oz	349	**142**	2.1	5
Cream cheese and salad	1 pack	156 g/5½ oz	294	**188**	4.7	4
Egg and ham	1 pack	262 g/9¼ oz	589	**225**	12.8	4
Egg and salad, mayonnaise, wholemeal bread	1 pack	180 g/6⅓ oz	257	**143**	4.9	7
Egg mayonnaise	1 pack	180 g/6⅓ oz	396	**220**	11.4	4
Egg, bacon and sausage	1 pack	249 g/8⅞ oz	655	**263**	13.2	4
Goats' cheese and chargrilled veg.	1 pack	214 g/7½ oz	481	**225**	9.2	5
Ham salad	1 pack	187 g/6⅗ oz	325	**174**	4.8	5
Houmous salad in flatbread	1 pack	180 g/6⅓ oz	319	**177**	6.2	4
Pork and apple sauce	1 pack	180 g/6⅓ oz	341	**190**	4.5	4

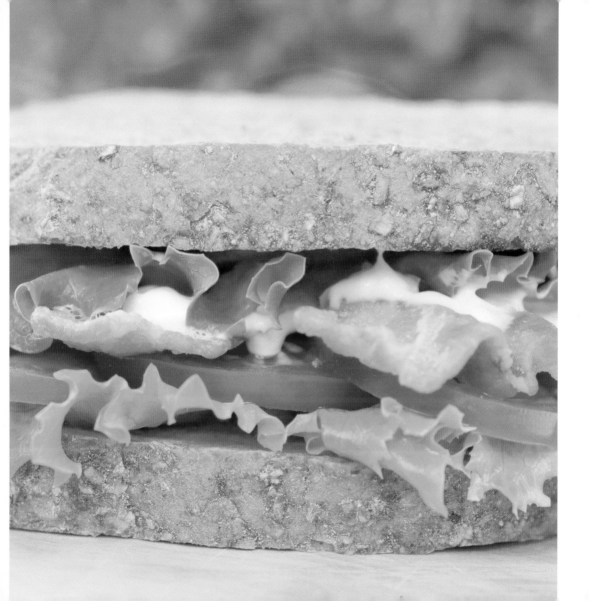

Counting Calories: Snacks, Confectionery & Desserts

	Typical portion	Typical portion size	Calories per portion	Calories per 100 g/ml	Fat per 100 g/ml	Health rating (1–10)
Prawn and smoked salmon	1 pack	225 g/8 oz	574	**255**	14.3	6
Prawn mayonnaise, oatmeal bread	1 pack	180 g/6⅓ oz	463	**257**	15.0	6
Salmon, cucumber and mayonnaise (deep fill)	1 pack	219 g/7⅔ oz	530	**242**	12.0	5
Spicy American, flatbread	1 pack	184 g/6½ oz	282	**153**	2.7	4
Tuna mayonnaise and cucumber	1 pack	225 g/8 oz	484	**215**	8.5	4

Rolls

All day breakfast	1	200 g/7 oz	528	**264**	12.0	3
Bacon and sausage	1	200 g/7 oz	630	**315**	27.7	3
Cheese and pickle	1	200 g/7 oz	528	**264**	10.0	3
Chicken salad	1	200 g/7 oz	298	**149**	2.0	5
Egg and tomato	1	200 g/7 oz	362	**181**	3.2	5
Egg mayonnaise	1	200 g/7 oz	390	**195**	6.9	5
Ham salad	1	200 g/7 oz	280	**140**	2.6	5
Roast chicken	1	200 g/7 oz	564	**282**	14.0	5
Roast pork and stuffing	1	200 g/7 oz	552	**276**	12.0	3
Smoked salmon	1	200 g/7 oz	304	**252**	11.3	5
Steak and onion	1	200 g/7 oz	410	**205**	7.0	3
Turkey and stuffing	1	200 g/7 oz	284	**142**	4.2	4

Panini

Bacon	1 pack	150 g/5 oz	273	**182**	6.6	4
Cheese	1 pack	150 g/5 oz	373	**249**	9.1	4
Ham and cheese	1 pack	223 g/7⅞ oz	557	**250**	11.7	4

	Typical portion	Typical portion size	Calories per portion	Calories per 100 g/ml	Fat per 100 g/ml	Health rating (1–10)
Mozzarella and tomato	1 pack	176 g/6⅕ oz	484	**275**	16.2	4
Tuna and sweetcorn	1 pack	200 g/7 oz	448	**224**	6.6	5
Bagels						
Cheese and jalapeño	1	115 g/4 oz	292	**254**	3.1	3
Chicken, lemon and watercress	1	153 g/5⅔ oz	329	**215**	4.1	4
Chicken, Louisiana-style	1	163 g/5½ oz	311	**191**	3.0	3
Cream cheese	1	120 g/4 oz	458	**352**	21.8	3
Ham, cream cheese and chives	1	160 g/5½ oz	320	**200**	4.4	3
Smoked salmon and cream cheese	1	155 g/5½ oz	434	**280**	12.2	4
Smoked salmon and soft cheese	1	155 g/5½ oz	338	**218**	6.0	4
Smoked salmon	1	140 g/5 oz	284	**203**	2.9	5
Tuna and sweetcorn	1	165 g/5½ oz	289	**175**	2.7	4
Tuna salad	1	170 g/6 oz	325	**191**	4.2	5
Turkey, pastrami and American mustard	1	146 g/5 oz	296	**203**	3.4	4
Baguettes						
Cheese and ham	½	190 g/6¾ oz	555	**292**	12.0	4
Cheese and onion	½	200 g/7 oz	732	**366**	17.6	4
Cheese and tomato	½	210 g/7⅓ oz	690	**329**	14.0	4
Chicken and mayonnaise	½	215 g/7½ oz	460	**214**	8.7	4
Chicken, bacon, salad and cheese	½	294 g/10⅓ oz	491	**167**	20.1	4
Egg and tomato	½	200 g/7 oz	420	**210**	7.6	5
Meatballs, sauce and cheese	½	319 g/11¼ oz	506	**158**	20.8	3

Counting Calories: Snacks, Confectionery & Desserts

	Typical portion	Typical portion size	Calories per portion	Calories per 100 g/ml	Fat per 100 g/ml	Health rating (1–10)
Mixed cheese and onion	½	200 g/7 oz	662	**331**	18.3	4
Steak strips, salad and melted cheese	½	247 g/8⅝ oz	332	**135**	8.9	4
Tuna, salad and light mayonnaise	½	247 g/8⅝ oz	398	**161**	17.7	5
Turkey and ham	½	215 g/7½ oz	462	**215**	5.1	5
Toasties						
All day breakfast	1 pack	174 g/6 oz	375	**215**	7.9	3
Cheese and ham	1 pack	136 g/4⅘ oz	706	**519**	29.7	3
Cheese on toast	1 slice	40 g/1½ oz	152	**380**	26.3	3
Melt, tuna	1 melt	100 g/3½ oz	285	**285**	17.0	3
Melt, cheesy fish	1 melt	100 g/3½ oz	123	**123**	6.6	3
Melt, salmon and broccoli	1 melt	100 g/3½ oz	93	**93**	3.3	3
Melt, vegetable and potato wedge	1 melt	100 g/3½ oz	451	**451**	23.0	3
Fajitas						
Beef	1 wrap	200 g/7 oz	340	**170**	4.7	4
Chicken	1 wrap	200 g/7 oz	500	**250**	2.3	4
Chicken with salsa and sour cream dip	1 wrap	200 g/7 oz	322	**161**	6.1	3
Tuna	1 wrap	200 g/7 oz	334	**167**	5.4	4
Vegetable	1 wrap	200 g/7 oz	256	**128**	5.0	4
Antipasti						
Antipasto, artichoke	1 dssp	50 g/2 oz	68	**135**	12.5	6
Antipasto, mixed mushroom	1 dssp	50 g/2 oz	49	**97**	9.0	6
Antipasto, mixed pepper	1 dssp	50 g/2 oz	63	**126**	8.4	6

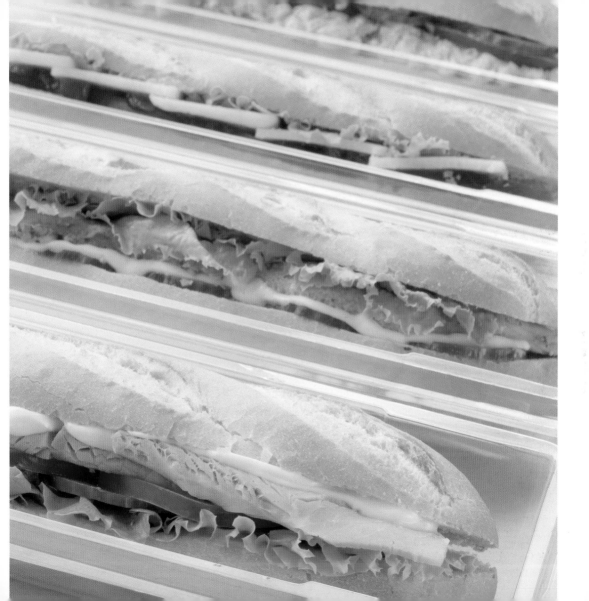

Counting Calories: Snacks, Confectionery & Desserts

	Typical portion	Typical portion size	Calories per portion	Calories per 100 g/ml	Fat per 100 g/ml	Health rating (1–10)
Antipasto, seafood	1 dssp	50 g/2 oz	80	**178**	11.6	6
Antipasto, sun-dried tomato	1 dssp	50 g/2 oz	116	**232**	16.8	6
Nibbles and Crisps						
Bombay mix	1 handful	30 g/1 oz	150	**503**	32.9	2
Breadsticks	4	20 g/¾ oz	78	**392**	8.4	2
Cheese puffs	1 bag	20 g/¾ oz	108	**542**	34.9	2
Cheese straws, home-made	1	41 g/1½ oz	173	**422**	30.7	3
Cheese straws, retail	1	11 g/⅖ oz	59	**535**	34.9	2
Corn snacks (e.g. Wotsits, etc.)	1 handful	30 g/1 oz	156	**519**	31.9	2
Popping corn	1 handful	30 g/1 oz	112	**375**	4.3	2
Popcorn, plain	1 handful	30 g/1 oz	178	**593**	42.8	2
Popcorn, salted	1 bag	75 g/3 oz	389	**519**	33.6	1
Popcorn, candied	1 handful	30 g/1 oz	144	**480**	20.0	2
Popcorn, butter toffee, microwave	1 bag	50 g/2 oz	252	**504**	30.0	1
Pork scratchings	1 pack	28 g/1 oz	180	**606**	46.0	1
Potato crisps, average	1 pack	28 g/1 oz	159	**530**	34.2	2
Potato crisps, average, reduced fat	1 pack	28 g/1 oz	138	**458**	21.5	2
Potato rings (e.g. Hula Hoops)	1 pack	28 g/1 oz	146	**523**	32.0	1
Pretzels, American style, salted	1 pack	50 g/2 oz	202	**403**	4.5	1
Tortilla chips	1 pack	35 g/1¼ oz	161	**459**	22.6	1
Yeast extract snacks (e.g. Twiglets), plain	1 bag	30 g/1 oz	117	**390**	10.8	1
Pot savouries (e.g. Pot Noodle), made up	1 pot	240 g/8½ oz	245	**103**	3.1	1

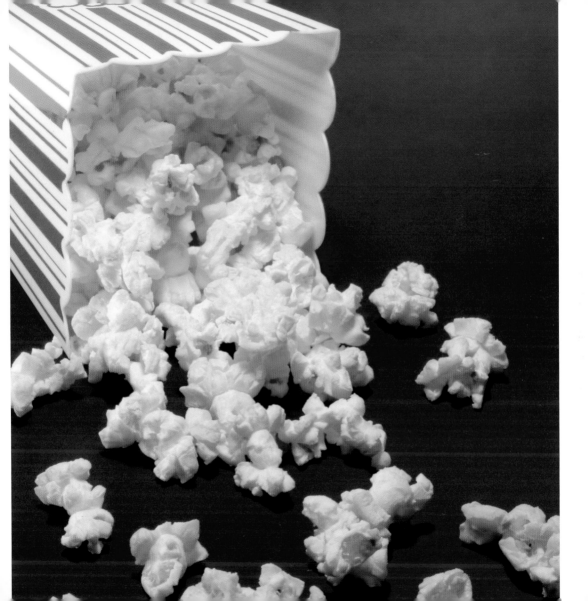

	Typical portion	Typical portion size	Calories per portion	Calories per 100 g/ml	Fat per 100 g/ml	Health rating (1–10)
Soups						
Beef and vegetable, canned	1 can	400 g/14 oz	212	**53**	1.0	5
Beef and vegetable, fresh	½ carton	300 g/11 oz	177	**59**	2.2	6
Bouillon, beef	½ can	210 g/7⅛ oz	153	**73**	0.5	5
Bouillon, chicken	½ can	210 g/7⅛ oz	154	**75**	3.0	5
Bouillon, fish	½ can	210 g/7⅛ oz	145	**69**	0.3	5
Bouillon, vegetable	½ can	210 g/7⅓ oz	211	**101**	0.3	5
Carrot and coriander, canned	1 can	415 g/14⅔ oz	170	**41**	1.5	5
Carrot and coriander, fresh	½ carton	300 g/11 oz	150	**50**	3.4	6
Chicken, condensed	½ can	210 g/7⅓ oz	179	**85**	5.8	4
Chicken, condensed, as served	½ can	210 g/7⅓ oz	91	**43**	2.9	4
Chicken, cream of, canned	1 can	415 g/14⅔ oz	240	**58**	3.8	4
Chicken, low calorie, canned	1 can	415 g/14⅔ oz	83	**20**	0.2	4
Consommé	½ can	210 g/7⅓ oz	26	**12**	0.0	5
Consommé, beef, canned	½ can	210 g/7⅓ oz	27	**13**	0.0	5
Gumbo, Cajun vegetable	1 bowl	400 g/14 oz	236	**59**	2.5	4
Gumbo, Louisiana chicken	1 bowl	400 g/14 oz	352	**88**	2.8	4
Minestrone, canned	1 can	415 g/14⅔ oz	129	**31**	0.5	4
Mushroom, cream of, canned	1 can	415 g/14⅔ oz	191	**46**	3.0	4
Oxtail, canned	1 can	415 g/14⅔ oz	183	**44**	1.7	4
Packet soup, average, dried	1 satchet	28 g/1 oz	32	**396**	14.3	2
P. soup, average, dried, made up	1 bowl	300 g/11 oz	192	**64**	2.3	2

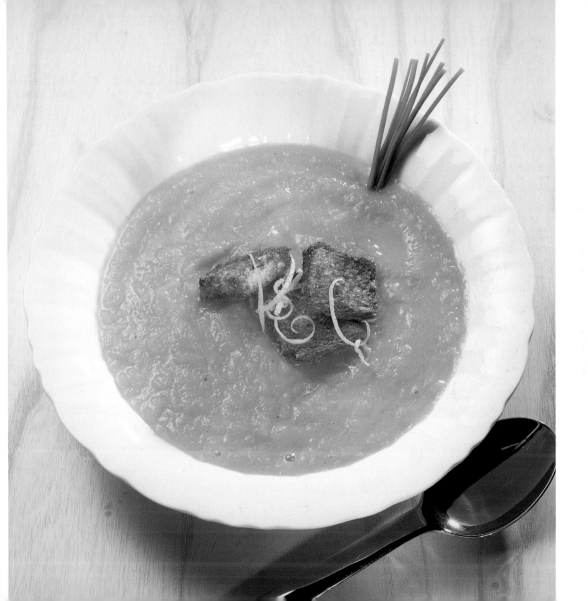

Counting Calories: Snacks, Confectionery & Desserts

	Typical portion	Typical portion size	Calories per portion	Calories per 100 g/ml	Fat per 100 g/ml	Health rating (1–10)
P. soup, chicken noodle, dried, made up	1 bowl	300 g/11 oz	57	**19**	0.3	2
P. soup, minestrone, dried, made up	1 bowl	300 g/11 oz	66	**22**	0.4	2
P. soup, tomato, dried, made up	1 bowl	300 g/11 oz	108	**36**	1.3	2
P. soup, vegetable, dried, made up	1 bowl	300 g/11 oz	66	**22**	0.3	2
Tomato, condensed	½ can	210 g/7⅓ oz	258	**123**	6.8	4
Tomato, condensed, made up	1 bowl	300 g/11 oz	186	**62**	3.4	4
Tomato, cream of, canned	½ can	210 g/7⅓ oz	210	**52**	3.0	4
Vegetable, canned	1 can	415 g/14⅔ oz	200	**48**	0.6	4

Ice Creams and Sorbets – *see also* pages 42–46, 152–54 and 226–32 for more desserts

	Typical portion	Typical portion size	Calories per portion	Calories per 100 g/ml	Fat per 100 g/ml	Health rating (1–10)
Ice cream, chocolate	1 scoop	50 g/2 oz	119	**238**	12.9	2
Ice cream, chocolate, premium	1 scoop	50 g/2 oz	143	**286**	18.7	3
Ice cream, strawberry	1 scoop	50 g/2 oz	93	**185**	9.3	3
Ice cream, strawberry, premium	1 scoop	50 g/2 oz	120	**241**	15.5	4
Ice cream, vanilla, dairy	1 scoop	50 g/2 oz	88	**177**	9.8	3
Ice cream, vanilla, dairy, premium	1 scoop	50 g/2 oz	108	**215**	15.1	4
Ice cream, vanilla, non-dairy	1 scoop	50 g/2 oz	76	**153**	7.8	3
Choc ice	1	80 g/3 oz	236	**295**	21.7	2
Choc ice, premium	1	60 g/2 oz	104	**340**	21.0	2
Chocolate nut sundae	1 pot	102 g/3⅗ oz	248	**243**	14.9	2
Cornetto-type ice cream cone	1	75 g/3 oz	213	**284**	17.8	2
Ice cream dessert/sundae	1 pot	90 g/3¼ oz	226	**251**	17.6	2
Ice cream dessert, viennetta-type	⅙	60 g/2 oz	183	**315**	20.9	2

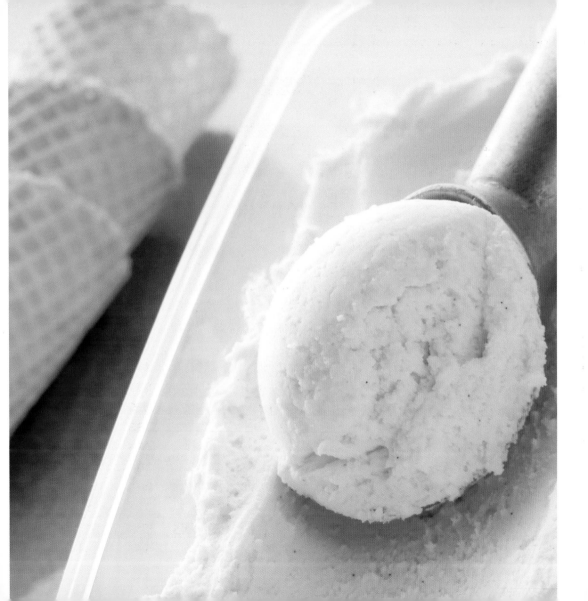

	Typical portion	Typical portion size	Calories per portion	Calories per 100 g/ml	Fat per 100 g/ml	Health rating (1–10)
Ice cream bar, choc. coated, family size	⅙	64 g/2½ oz	202	**311**	23.3	2
Ice cream roll (Arctic roll)	¼	60 g/2 oz	138	**230**	8.6	2
Lolly, ice cream, chocolate coated	1	75 g/3 oz	215	**287**	19.0	2
Lolly, ice cream, chocolate, premium	1	75 g/3 oz	247	**331**	23.8	3
Lolly, fruit and ice cream	1	75 g/3 oz	83	**110**	3.0	3
Lolly, fruit	1	75 g/3 oz	53	**70**	0.1	3
Lolly, with real fruit juice	1	56 g/2 oz	41	**73**	0.3	4
Sorbet, fruit	1 scoop	50 g/2 oz	45	**97**	0.3	4
Sorbet, fruit, premium	1 scoop	50 g/2/ oz	60	**119**	0.2	4
Ice cream wafers	1	10 g/¼ oz	35	**342**	0.7	2
Whipped ice cream (e.g. McFlurry), choc. mint	1 tub	204 g/7⅕ oz	381	**187**	5.4	2
Whipped ice cream, choc. caramel	1 tub	204 g/7⅕ oz	385	**187**	6.3	2
Whipped ice cream, jam biscuit	1 tub	128 g/4½ oz	256	**200**	6.4	2
Whipped ice cream, toffee swirl	1 tub	204 g/7 oz	400	**194**	6.0	2

Puddings and Chilled Desserts

Baklava	1 bag	50 g/2 oz	194	**393**	21.0	2
Banana split, with cream and sauce	1 banana	240 g/8½ oz	463	**193**	13.0	4
Cheesecake, frozen	1 slice	80 g/3 oz	232	**294**	16.2	2
Cheesecake, fruit, individual	1	90 g/3¼ oz	238	**264**	12.3	2
Chocolate dairy desserts	1	90 g/3¼ oz	193	**214**	10.7	2
Crepe, chocolate-filled	1	50 g/2 oz	219	**437**	18.1	3
Crumble, fruit	2 tbsp	115 g/4 oz	252	**219**	8.3	4

	Typical portion	Typical portion size	Calories per portion	Calories per 100 g/ml	Fat per 100 g/ml	Health rating (1–10)
Crumble, fruit, wholemeal	2 tbsp	115 g/4 oz	224	**195**	7.4	5
Crumble, rhubarb	¼ pack	150 g/5 oz	311	**208**	9.2	4
Jelly, made with water	2 tbsp	56 g/2 oz	34	**61**	0.0	2
Meringue	1	30 g/1 oz	114	**381**	0.0	3
Meringue, with cream	1	85 g/3 oz	280	**330**	24.2	2
Pancake, scotch	1	35 g/1¼ oz	112	**280**	4.0	3
Pancake, scotch, low fat	1	35 g/1¼ oz	109	**272**	2.2	4
Pancake, sweet, made with skimmed milk	1	34 g/1⅕ oz	95	**280**	13.8	4
Pancake, sweet, made with whole milk	1	34 g/1⅕ oz	103	**302**	16.3	4
Pavlova, with fruit and cream	3 tbsp	75 g/3 oz	216	**288**	13.2	4
Pie, apple	1 slice	75 g/3 oz	191	**255**	11.0	3
Pie, apple and blackberry	1 slice	75 g/3 oz	209	**279**	11.9	3
Pie, apple, deep filled	1 slice	75 g/3 oz	205	**273**	12.8	3
Pie, apple, puff pastry	1 slice	75 g/3 oz	188	**250**	12.7	3
Pie, apricot	1 slice₄	75 g/3 oz	233	**311**	10.0	3
Pie, banoffee	1 slice	75 g/3 oz	240	**319**	20.0	2
Pie, blackcurrant	1 slice	75 g/3 oz	218	**290**	10.1	3
Pie, fruit, individual	1	35 g/1¼ oz	125	**356**	14.0	2
Pie, fruit, one crust	1 slice	75 g/3 oz	143	**190**	8.2	4
Pie, fruit, wholemeal, one crust	1 slice	75 g/3 oz	138	**185**	8.3	5
Pie, fruit, wholemeal, pastry top and bottom	1 slice	75 g/3 oz	190	**253**	13.8	4
Pie, lemon meringue	2 tbsp	65 g/2½ oz	164	**251**	8.5	3

Counting Calories: Snacks, Confectionery & Desserts

	Typical portion	Typical portion size	Calories per portion	Calories per 100 g/ml	Fat per 100 g/ml	Health rating (1–10)
Pie, Mississippi mud	1 slice	75 g/3 oz	288	**384**	25.6	2
Profiteroles, with sauce	4	75 g/3 oz	269	**359**	23.9	2
Pudding, apple and custard	2 tbsp	115 g/4 oz	132	**115**	1.9	4
Pudding, bread	2 tbsp	115 g/4 oz	332	**289**	9.5	3
Pudding, Christmas	2 tbsp	115 g/4 oz	379	**329**	11.8	4
Pudding, Christmas, nut and alcohol free	2 tbsp	50 g/2 oz	129	**258**	2.7	5
Pudding, Christmas, rich fruit w/brandy	2 tbsp	50 g/2 oz	153	**305**	9.7	4
Pudding, Christmas, wheat and gluten free	2 tbsp	50 g/2 oz	149	**295**	7.1	5
Pudding, Queen of Puddings	2 tbsp	115 g/4 oz	181	**213**	7.8	4
Pudding, rice, canned	½ can	212 g/7½ oz	180	**85**	1.3	4
Pudding, rice, canned, low fat	½ can	212 g/7½ oz	151	**71**	0.8	4
Pudding, sticky toffee, with custard	2 tbsp	115 g/4 oz	306	**235**	8.0	2
Pudding, suet	1	100 g/3½ oz	335	**335**	18.3	1
Roly-poly, jam	3 tbsp	80 g/3 oz	287	**359**	14.2	2
Roly-poly, jam and custard	3 tbsp	80 g/3 oz	188	**235**	8.0	2
Sorbet, fruit	1 pot	100 g/3½ oz	120	**120**	0.0	5
Sponge pudding, canned	2 tbsp	115 g/4 oz	292	**265**	9.1	2
Spotted dick	1 pudding	110 g/4 oz	346	**315**	11.7	2
Strudel, apple	1 slice	65 g/2½ oz	184	**283**	15.4	2
Tart, apricot lattice	1 slice	65 g/2½ oz	174	**267**	16.0	4
Tart, Bakewell	1 slice	65 g/2½ oz	299	**460**	26.7	3
Tart, frangipane, chocolate	1 slice	65 g/2½ oz	178	**274**	15.5	3

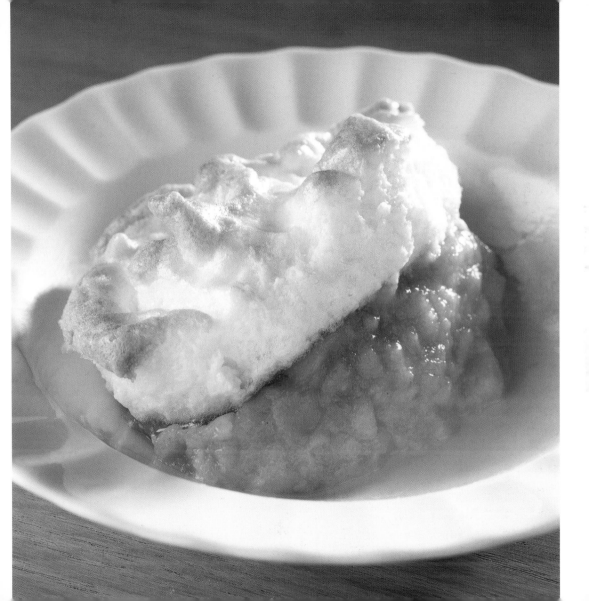

Counting Calories: Snacks, Confectionery & Desserts

	Typical portion	Typical portion size	Calories per portion	Calories per 100 g/ml	Fat per 100 g/ml	Health rating (1–10)
Tart, jam	1 slice	65 g/2½ oz	247	**380**	14.9	3
Tart, treacle	1 slice	65 g/2½ oz	247	**379**	14.2	3
Tarte au citron	1 slice	65 g/2½ oz	211	**325**	18.1	3
Tarte aux cerises	1 slice	65 g/2½ oz	146	**225**	18.2	3
Tarte tatin	1 slice	65 g/2½ oz	132	**203**	6.7	3
Tiramisu	2 tbsp	60 g/2 oz	148	**246**	12.4	1
Tiramisu, healthy range	2 tbsp	60 g/2 oz	140	**156**	2.7	2
Torte, chocolate	1 slice	80 g/3 oz	177	**221**	10.5	3
Torte, chocolate orange and almond	1 slice	80 g/3 oz	336	**420**	30.5	2
Torte, chocolate truffle	1 slice	80 g/3 oz	240	**309**	17.3	2
Torte, fruit	1 slice	80 g/3 oz	206	**258**	15.5	2
Torte, lemon and mango	1 slice	80 g/3 oz	142	**177**	3.0	2
Torte, raspberry	1 slice	80 g/3 oz	138	**172**	7.4	3
Trifle mix, dry	1 packet	35 g/1¼ oz	148	**425**	10.5	2
Trifle, average	2 tbsp	56 g/2 oz	90	**160**	6.3	3
Trifle, Black Forest, healthy range	2 tbsp	56 g/2 oz	77	**137**	4.5	3
Trifle, chocolate	2 tbsp	56 g/2 oz	140	**250**	15.2	2
Trifle, fruit	2 tbsp	56 g/2 oz	91	**164**	9.0	2
Trifle, individual	1	125 g/4 oz	208	**166**	8.1	3
Trifle, sherry	2 tbsp	56 g/2 oz	98	**175**	9.1	2
Turnover, apple	1	88 g/3⅛ oz	304	**346**	25.9	2
Turnover, apple, with dairy cream	1	92 g/3¼ oz	349	**380**	25.9	2

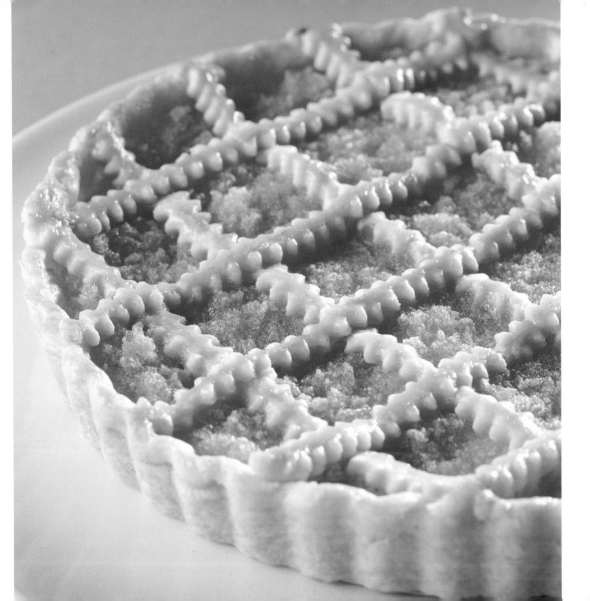

	Typical portion	Typical portion size	Calories per portion	Calories per 100 g/ml	Fat per 100 g/ml	Health rating (1–10)
Turnover, mincemeat, with cream	1	88 g/3⅑ oz	307	**405**	26.9	2
Turnover, raspberry, with cream	1	92 g/3¼ oz	378	**411**	23.0	2
Confectionery and Sweet Snacks						
Caramels, chocolate covered	6	66 g/2½ oz	307	**465**	21.7	2
Chocolate bar (e.g. Mars)	1	100/3½ oz	453	**453**	18.3	2
Chocolate bar (e.g. Milky Way)	1	26 g/1 oz	116	**445**	16.7	2
Chocolate bar (e.g. Snickers)	1	64 g/2½ oz	319	**497**	27.8	2
Chocolate bar, coconut	1 pack	57 g/2 oz	267	**469**	26.3	2
Chocolate biscuit bars (e.g. Twix)	1 finger	29 g/1 oz	142	**492**	24.1	2
Chocolate egg, Easter, with buttons	¼	50 g/2 oz	133	**530**	30.1	2
Chocolate egg, Easter, dark	¼	90 g/3¼ oz	472	**525**	37.4	4
Chocolate egg, Easter, honeycomb	¼	30 g/1 oz	158	**525**	30.0	1
Chocolate egg, Easter, white	¼	90 g/3¼ oz	487	**544**	30.3	2
Chocolate egg, fondant-filled (e.g. Creme Egg)	1	39 g/1⅜ oz	174	**445**	16.0	2
Chocolate egg, mini	1	11 g/⅖ oz	50	**445**	16.4	2
Chocolate wafers (e.g. Kit Kat)	2 fingers	21 g/¾ oz	105	**500**	26.0	2
Chocolate, milk	1 bar	50 g/2 oz	260	**520**	30.7	3
Chocolate, plain	1 bar	50 g/2 oz	255	**510**	28.0	4
Chocolate, white	1 bar	50 g/2 oz	265	**529**	30.9	2
Chocolate, fancy/filled	1 bar	50 g/2 oz	224	**447**	21.3	2
Dolly mixtures	1 pack	100 g/3½ oz	376	**376**	1.5	2
Fudge, all butter	1 bag	100 g/3½ oz	429	**429**	14.5	1

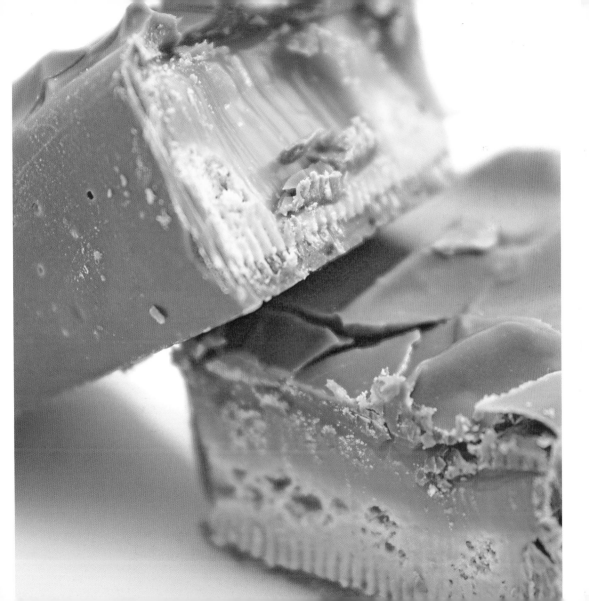

Counting Calories: Snacks, Confectionery & Desserts

	Typical portion	Typical portion size	Calories per portion	Calories per 100 g/ml	Fat per 100 g/ml	Health rating (1–10)
Fudge, cherry and almond	1 bag	100 g/3½ oz	464	**464**	19.1	1
Fudge, chocolate	1 bag	100 g/3½ oz	459	**459**	19.1	1
Fudge, clotted cream	1 bag	100 g/3½ oz	474	**474**	22.1	1
Fudge, double chocolate	1 bag	100 g/3½ oz	470	**470**	21.0	1
Fudge, vanilla	1 bag	100 g/3½ oz	465	**465**	21.9	1
Gums, American, hard	1 sweet	6 g/⅕ oz	22	**360**	0.1	2
Gums, milk bottles	2	6 g/⅕ oz	21	**353**	1.6	2
Gums/jellies, fruit	1 packet	35 g/1¼ oz	114	**324**	0.0	2
Halva	1 sweet	28 g/1 oz	107	**381**	13.2	2
Liquorice allsorts	1 handful	50 g/2 oz	175	**349**	5.2	3
Marshmallows	6	42 g/1½ oz	138	**327**	0.0	2
Marzipan, dark chocolate covered	1 bar	46 g/1⅝ oz	206	**448**	17.4	3
Mint creams	1	12 g/³⁄₇ oz	57	**477**	23.8	1
Mint humbugs	1	6 g/⅕ oz	20	**340**	4.4	1
Mint imperials	1	3 g/⅑ oz	12	**391**	0.0	1
Mints, soft	1	5 g/⅙ oz	18	**355**	0.0	1
Mints, after dinner	1	7 g/¼ oz	32	**456**	21.2	1
Mints, butter (mintoes)	1	7 g/¼ oz	27	**391**	6.8	1
Mints, clear	1	6 g/⅕ oz	24	**395**	0.0	1
Mints, Everton	1	5 g/⅙ oz	21	**410**	4.0	1
Pastilles, fruit	1 packet	50 g/2 oz	164	**327**	0.0	2
Peanut brittle	2 pieces	32 g/1⅛ oz	163	**509**	26.9	2

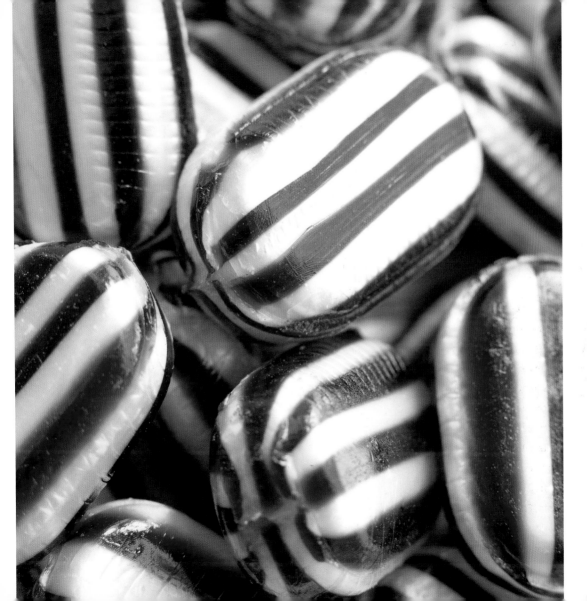

Counting Calories: Snacks, Confectionery & Desserts

	Typical portion	Typical portion size	Calories per portion	Calories per 100 g/ml	Fat per 100 g/ml	Health rating (1–10)
Peppermints	4	26 g/1 oz	102	**393**	0.7	2
Sherbert sweets	4	32 g/1⅛ oz	114	**355**	0.0	2
Sugar-coated sweets (e.g. Smarties)	1 tube	40 g/1½ oz	183	**456**	17.5	2
Sweets, boiled	4	32 g/1⅛ oz	105	**327**	0.0	2
Sweets, chewy	1 packet	50 g/2 oz	190	**381**	5.6	2
Toffees, mixed	4	32 g/1⅛ oz	136	**426**	18.6	2
Turkish delight, assorted flavours	1 pack	30 g/1 oz	110	**366**	0.1	2
Turkish delight, dark chocolate coating	1 chocolate	10 g/¼ oz	39	**390**	11.0	2
Turkish delight, milk chocolate coating	1 pack	55 g/2 oz	220	**400**	8.5	2

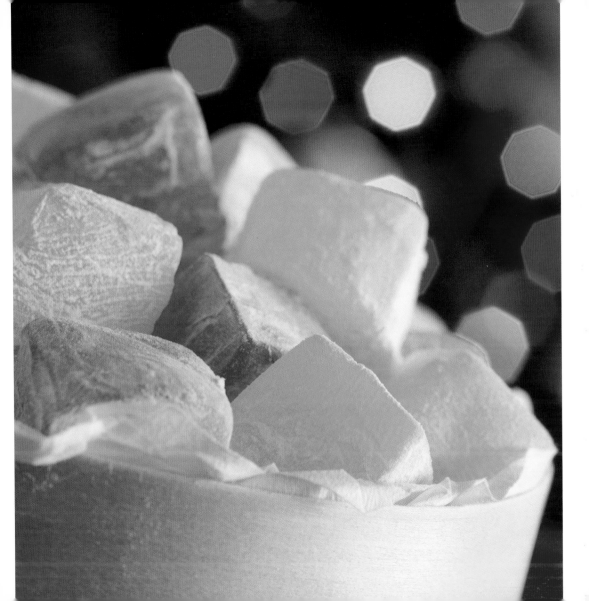

Takeaway & Convenience Food

	Typical portion	Typical portion size	Calories per portion	Calories per 100 g/ml	Fat per 100 g/ml	Health rating (1–10)
Oriental and Southeast Asian						
Beansprouts, fried	½ pack	200 g/7 oz	122	**61**	5.7	2
Beef in black bean sauce	1 pack	386 g/13⅗ oz	432	**112**	4.3	4
Chicken and cashew nuts	½ pack	200 g/7 oz	178	**89**	4.0	4
Chicken balls	½ pack	200 g/7 oz	560	**280**	13.6	2
Chow mein, beef	1 pack	225 g/8 oz	306	**136**	6.0	3
Chow mein, chicken	1 pack	200 g/7 oz	294	**147**	7.2	3
Duck, aromatic, crispy	2 slices	140 g/5 oz	396	**283**	15.0	2
Duck, arom., crispy and pancake w/hoisin sauce	1 piece	40 g/1½ oz	100	**250**	10.6	2
Egg fu yung	3 tbsp	80 g/3 oz	191	**239**	20.6	2
Fish balls, steamed	4	100 g/3½ oz	74	**74**	0.5	4
Laksa, chicken	1 bowl	300 ml/10 fl oz	240	**80**	2.2	3
Laksa, Thai noodle, with chicken	1 bowl	300 ml/10 fl oz	345	**115**	5.4	3
Nasi Goreng, Indonesian	½ pack	180 g/6⅓ oz	389	**216**	6.3	4
Pork Char Sui in Cantonese sauce	½ pack	200 g/7 oz	346	**173**	2.2	2
Pork Char Sui with chicken and egg-fried rice	½ pack	200 g/7 oz	268	**134**	3.6	3
Prawn crackers	1 handful	35 g/1¼ oz	199	**570**	39.0	2
Rice, egg-fried	3 tbsp	150 g/5 oz	315	**210**	7.0	2
Rice, special fried	½ packet	150 g/5 oz	308	**205**	7.8	3

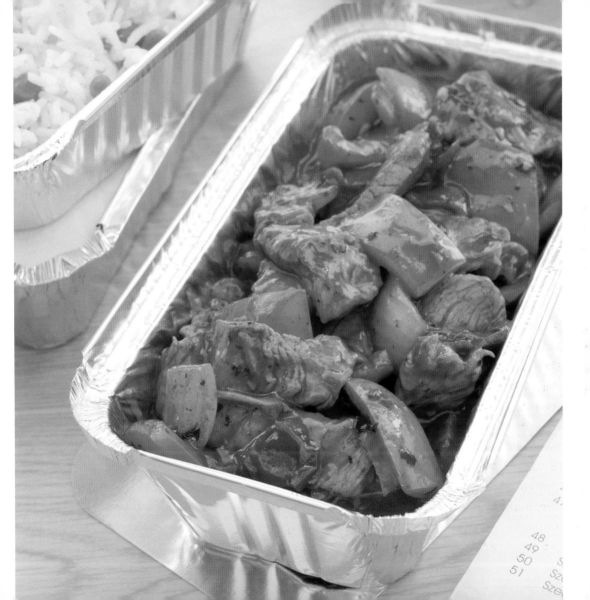

Counting Calories: Takeaway & Convenience Food

	Typical portion	Typical portion size	Calories per portion	Calories per 100 g/ml	Fat per 100 g/ml	Health rating (1–10)
Rice, sticky, Thai	3 tbsp	150 g/5 oz	195	**130**	1.8	2
Rice, sweet-and-sour	3 tbsp	150 g/5 oz	156	**104**	0.6	4
Satay, chicken, takeaway	2 pieces	90 g/3¼ oz	172	**191**	10.3	3
Spring rolls, meat	1	70 g/3½ oz	170	**242**	16.4	2
Spring rolls, vegetable	1	70 g/3½ oz	155	**221**	11.3	3
Stir-fry, beef, with green peppers	1 bowl	225 g/8 oz	318	**141**	8.0	6
Stir-fry, chicken, rice and veg.; frozen, reheated	1 pack	225 g/8 oz	297	**132**	4.6	5
Stir-fry, vegetable, takeaway	1 pack	200 g/7 oz	104	**52**	4.1	4
Sweet-and-sour chicken	1 pack	400 g/14 oz	776	**194**	10.0	3
Sweet-and-sour pork	½ pack	165 g/5½ oz	546	**331**	5.8	2
Sweet-and-sour pork, home-made	1 bowl	225 g/8 oz	398	**177**	8.6	4
Szechuan prawns with vegetables	1 pack	200 g/7 oz	166	**83**	4.7	5

Indian

	Typical portion	Typical portion size	Calories per portion	Calories per 100 g/ml	Fat per 100 g/ml	Health rating (1–10)
Balti bhuna, lamb	½ pack	200 g/7 oz	180	**90**	3.7	4
Balti, chicken	½ pack	175 g/6 oz	245	**140**	8.7	4
Balti, chicken, with rice, diet	½ pack	165 g/5½ oz	127	**77**	1.7	5
Balti, vegetable, with rice	½ pack	225 g/8 oz	189	**84**	1.6	4
Bhaji, aubergine and potato	1	35 g/1¼ oz	46	**130**	8.8	4
Bhaji, cauliflower	1	35 g/1¼ oz	75	**214**	20.5	4
Bhaji, mushroom	1	35 g/1¼ oz	58	**166**	16.1	3
Bhaji, okra	1	35 g/1¼ oz	33	**95**	6.4	3
Bhaji, onion	1	35 g/1¼ oz	71	**203**	9.8	3

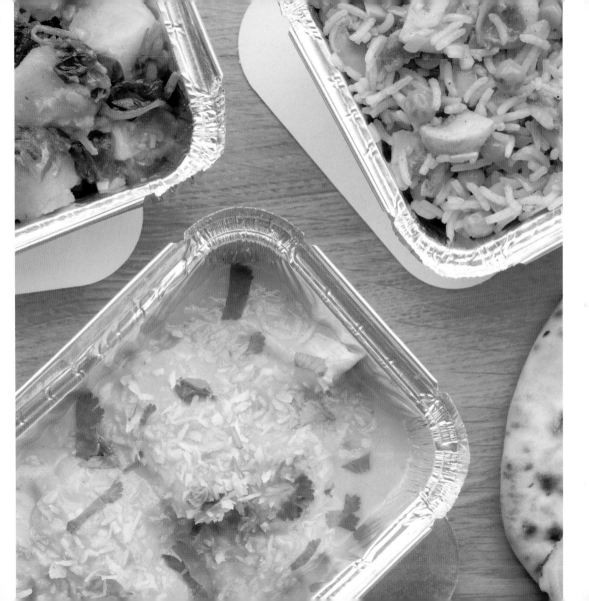

Counting Calories: Takeaway & Convenience Food

	Typical portion	Typical portion size	Calories per portion	Calories per 100 g/ml	Fat per 100 g/ml	Health rating (1–10)
Bhaji, potato and onion	1	35 g/1¼ oz	56	**160**	10.1	3
Bhaji, potato and spinach	1	35 g/1¼ oz	67	**191**	14.1	3
Bhaji, vegetable	1	35 g/1¼ oz	74	**212**	18.5	3
Biryani, chicken	1 pack	370 g/13 oz	289	**78**	0.5	4
Biryani, chicken tikka	1 pack	400 g/14 oz	436	**109**	1.9	4
Biryani, chicken tikka, with rice	1 pack	375 g/13 oz	484	**129**	4.3	4
Biryani, vegetable, with rice	1 pack	370 g/13 oz	481	**130**	5.5	4
Bombay potato	½ pack	200 g/7 oz	202	**101**	5.2	4
Channa masala	1 pack	225 g/8 oz	360	**160**	10.5	4
Curry, beef, chilled/frozen, reheated	1 pack	225 g/8 oz	307	**137**	6.6	3
Curry, beef, chilled/frozen, with rice, reheated	1 pack	300 g/11 oz	393	**131**	3.9	3
Curry, beef, ch./fr., with rice, reduced fat, reheated	1 pack	300 g/11 oz	429	**143**	7.1	3
Curry, chickpea dhal	1 pack	225 g/8 oz	338	**154**	6.1	5
Curry, chicken	1 pack	200 g/7 oz	290	**145**	9.8	3
Curry, chicken, chilled/frozen, with rice, reheated	1 pack	300 g/11 oz	411	**137**	5.0	3
Curry, chicken, made with canned curry sauce	1 bowl	300 g/11 oz	450	**150**	6.5	3
Curry, fish, Bangladeshi	1 pack	200 g/7 oz	254	**127**	8.0	4
Curry, lamb, made with canned curry sauce	1 bowl	300 g/11 oz	747	**249**	18.9	2
Curry, prawn	1 pack	200 g/7 oz	234	**117**	8.5	4
Curry, vegetable, with rice	1 bowl	300 g/11 oz	306	**102**	3.0	5
Jalfrezi, chicken	½ pack	200 g/7 oz	238	**119**	6.5	4
Keema, lamb	1 pack	225 g/8 oz	528	**176**	13.4	4

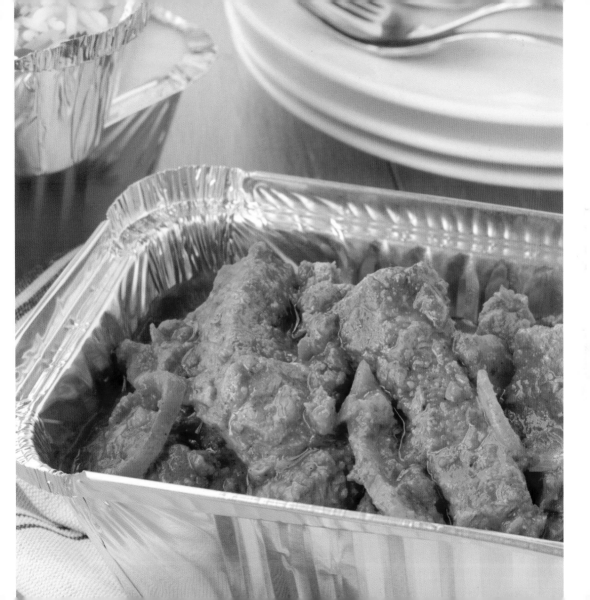

Counting Calories: Takeaway & Convenience Food

	Typical portion	Typical portion size	Calories per portion	Calories per 100 g/ml	Fat per 100 g/ml	Health rating (1–10)
Korma, chicken	½ pack	200 g/7 oz	332	**166**	10.3	3
Madras sauce, beef in	1 pack	400 g/14 oz	344	**86**	3.6	3
Pakora, chicken tikka	1	50 g/2 oz	100	**199**	11.0	4
Pakora, potato and spinach	1	50 g/2 oz	120	**240**	16.5	4
Pakora, vegetable	1	50 g/2 oz	133	**265**	18.1	4
Pasanda, chicken	½ pack	140 g/5 oz	258	**184**	12.4	4
Samosa, chicken tikka	1	50 g/2 oz	119	**119**	12.9	2
Samosa, lamb	1	50 g/2 oz	144	**144**	15.7	2
Samosa, vegetable	½ pack	100 g/3½ oz	252	**252**	13.2	2
Tandoori, chicken, chilled, reheated	1 pack	300 g/11 oz	642	**214**	10.8	5
Tikka masala, chicken	1 pack	225/8 oz	354	**157**	10.6	4

Burgers and Fried Food – *see also* pages 94–100 and 130–40 for other meat and vegetable products

	Typical portion	Typical portion size	Calories per portion	Calories per 100 g/ml	Fat per 100 g/ml	Health rating (1–10)
(Beef) hamburger	1	100 g/3½ oz	243	**243**	9.6	3
(Beef) hamburger, 'deluxe', with bacon	1	274 g/9⅔ oz	689	**252**	14.0	3
(Beef) hamburger, Big Mac style	1	217 g/7⅔ oz	495	**228**	10.7	3
(Beef) cheeseburger	1	115 g/4 oz	300	**259**	11.8	3
(Beef) cheeseburger with bacon	1	127 g/4½ oz	336	**264**	12.0	2
(Beef) cheeseburger, double	1	169 g/6 oz	446	**263**	13.0	3
(Beef) cheeseburger, quarter-pounder	1	200 g/7 oz	500	**250**	13.0	3
Big breakfast	1 pack	264 g/9⅓ oz	595	**225**	13.0	2
Burger, vegetarian, 'deluxe'	1	181 g/6⅜ oz	411	**227**	9.0	2
Butty, bacon	1	126 g/4⅖ oz	391	**310**	13.0	3

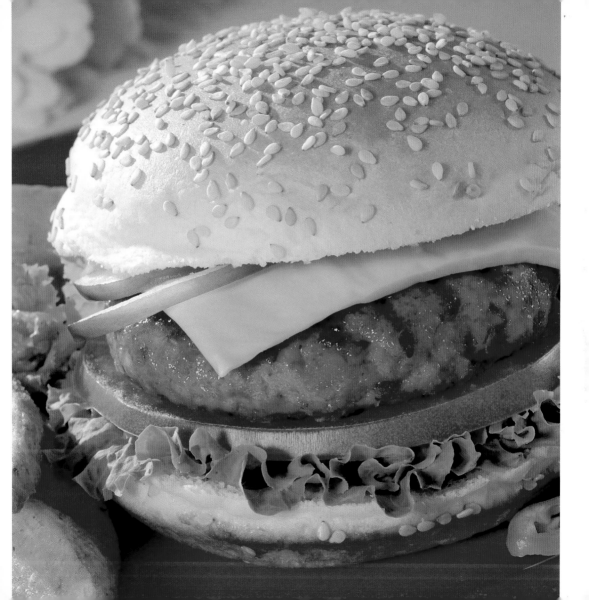

Counting Calories: Takeaway & Convenience Food

	Typical portion	Typical portion size	Calories per portion	Calories per 100 g/ml	Fat per 100 g/ml	Health rating (1–10)
Butty, bacon and egg	1	176 g/6 oz	475	**270**	13.0	3
Butty, egg and cheese	1	164 g/5½ oz	454	**277**	14.0	2
Butty, sausage	1	193 g/6⅘ oz	587	**304**	17.0	3
Butty, sausage and egg	1	243 g/8 4/7 oz	671	**276**	16.0	2
Chicken breast, southern fried	1	137 g/4⅚ oz	285	**207**	9.7	3
Chicken burger	1	210 g/7⅓ oz	560	**267**	10.8	2
Chicken burger, mini/kids	1	114 g/4 oz	253	**222**	5.6	2
Chicken drumsticks	1	80 g/3 oz	233	**291**	17.9	2
Chicken drumsticks, southern fried	1	95 g/3⅓ oz	161	**170**	10.0	2
Chicken fillet tower burger	1	163 g/5½ oz	617	**378**	12.9	1
Chicken nuggets	6	100 g/3½ oz	265	**265**	13.0	2
Chicken strips, southern fried	1	46 g/1⅝ oz	112	**243**	11.7	2
Chicken thighs, southern fried	1	134 g/4 5/7 oz	218	**162**	10.6	3
Chicken wings, southern fried	1	17 g/⅗ oz	150	**862**	45.4	2
Fillet o' fish	1 burger	147 g/5 oz	341	**232**	11.0	3
Fish (cod) in batter, fried in blended oil	1 fillet	300 g/11 oz	741	**247**	15.4	3
Fish (haddock) in batter	1 fillet	300 g/11 oz	684	**228**	12.2	3
Fish (hoki) steaks in batter	1	150 g/5 oz	390	**260**	13.9	3
Fish (lemon sole) goujons, fried in blended oil	6	175 g/6 oz	655	**374**	28.7	2
Fish (plaice) goujons, fried in blended oil	6	175 g/6 oz	745	**426**	32.3	2
Fish (plaice) in batter, fried in blended oil	1 fillet	300 g/11 oz	771	**257**	16.8	3
Fish (plaice) in crumbs, fried in blended oil	1 fillet	175 g/6 oz	399	**228**	13.7	4

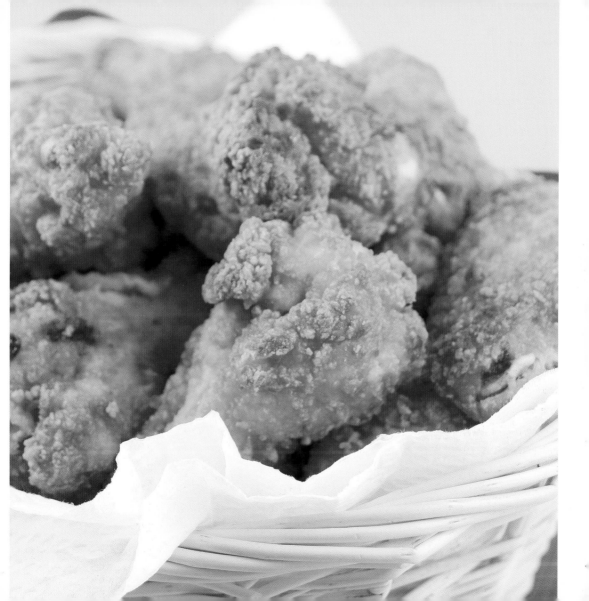

Counting Calories: Takeaway & Convenience Food

	Typical portion	Typical portion size	Calories per portion	Calories per 100 g/ml	Fat per 100 g/ml	Health rating (1–10)
Fish (red snapper), fried in blended oil	1 fillet	100 g/3½ oz	126	**126**	3.1	3
Fish (rock salmon) in batter, fried in blended oil	1 fillet	300 g/11 oz	885	**295**	21.9	3
Fish (skate) in batter, fried in blended oil	1 fillet	300 g/11 oz	504	**168**	10.1	3
Fish (whitebait), in flour, fried	1 bowl	150 g/5 oz	787	**525**	47.5	2
Fish (whiting) in crumbs, fried in blended oil	1 fillet	175 g/6 oz	335	**191**	10.3	3
Fish and chips, breaded, frozen, ready to cook	1 pack	350 g/12 oz	560	**160**	5.3	3
Fish and chips, takeaway	1 medium	350 g/12 oz	764	**218**	12.2	4
Hash browns	1 piece	57 g/2 oz	140	**246**	14.0	2
Hot dog/frankfurter in a bun, with cheese	1	172 g/6 oz	432	**251**	14.1	2
Onion rings, battered	5	100 g/3½ oz	219	**219**	10.0	3
Potato cake, fried	1	70 g/2½ oz	166	**237**	9.0	2
Potato fries, large	1 tub	160 g/5½ oz	460	**288**	14.0	2
Potato fries, regular	1 tub	114 g/4 oz	330	**298**	14.0	2
Potato fries, small	1 tub	79 g/3 oz	228	**288**	14.0	2
Potato wedges	1 tub	180 g/6⅓ oz	373	**207**	9.6	2
Prawns in batter, crisp	1 pack	160 g/5½ oz	350	**219**	12.7	2
Saveloy, unbattered, takeaway	1	130 g/4½ oz	225	**296**	22.3	1
Scampi, in breadcr., frozen, fried in blended oil	10	75 g/3 oz	178	**237**	13.6	3
Squid, in batter, fried in blended oil	1 bowl	125 g/4 oz	247	**195**	10.0	2
Kebabs						
Doner, in pitta bread, with salad	1	400 g/14 oz	1020	**255**	16.2	1
Doner, meat only	1 tray	200 g/7 oz	754	**377**	31.4	1

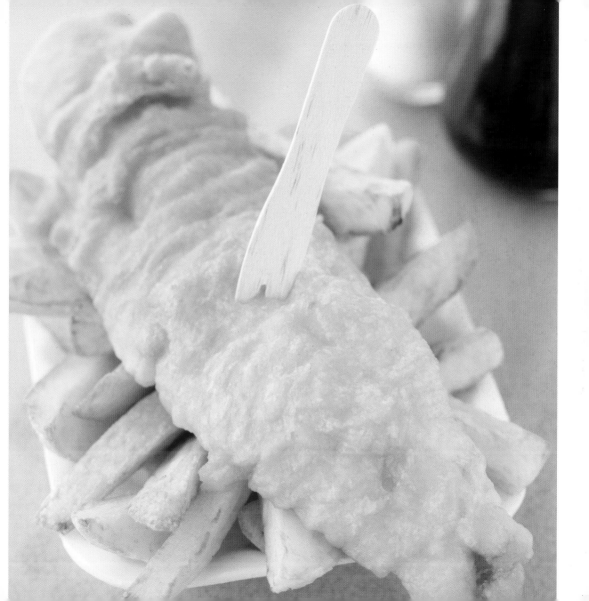

Counting Calories: Takeaway & Convenience Food

	Typical portion	Typical portion size	Calories per portion	Calories per 100 g/ml	Fat per 100 g/ml	Health rating (1–10)
Kebab, average, chicken	1 kebab	100 g/3½ oz	113	**113**	3.2	5
Kebab, average, vegetable	1 kebab	100 g/3½ oz	36	**36**	0.5	5
Shish, beef	1 kebab	100 g/3½ oz	225	**225**	17.3	2
Shish, chicken	1 kebab	100 g/3½ oz	125	**125**	2.1	3
Shish, lamb	1 kebab	100 g/3½ oz	210	**210**	13.3	2
Shish, pork	1 kebab	100 g/3½ oz	158	**158**	5.4	3
Shish, salmon	1 kebab	100 g/3½ oz	118	**118**	2.9	3
Pizzas						
American hot, 12"	½	264 g/9⅓ oz	562	**213**	7.5	3
American hot, 5", frozen	1	170 g/6 oz	445	**262**	11.8	3
Bacon and mushroom	½	185 g/6½ oz	370	**200**	6.4	3
Cajun chicken	½	165 g/5½ oz	363	**220**	3.6	3
Cheese and tomato, average	1	300 g/11 oz	711	**237**	11.8	3
Cheese and tomato (Margherita)	1 slice	88 g/3⅛ oz	172	**195**	3.6	3
Cheese and tomato, thin and crispy	1	155 g/5½ oz	355	**229**	7.8	3
Chicken and bacon, carbonara, thin crust	½	246 g/8⅔ oz	578	**235**	7.0	3
Chicken and chargrilled vegetable	½	184 g/6½ oz	383	**208**	8.0	3
Chicken, pesto and red peppers	½	192 g/6⅞ oz	471	**245**	9.7	3
Chicken, thin and crispy, frozen	½	157 g/5½ oz	469	**299**	12.7	3
Chilli beef	½	198 g/7 oz	396	**200**	5.8	3
Farmhouse, thin, medium	1 slice	88 g/3⅛ oz	244	**277**	12.2	3
Four cheese	½	230 g/8⅛ oz	575	**250**	9.2	3

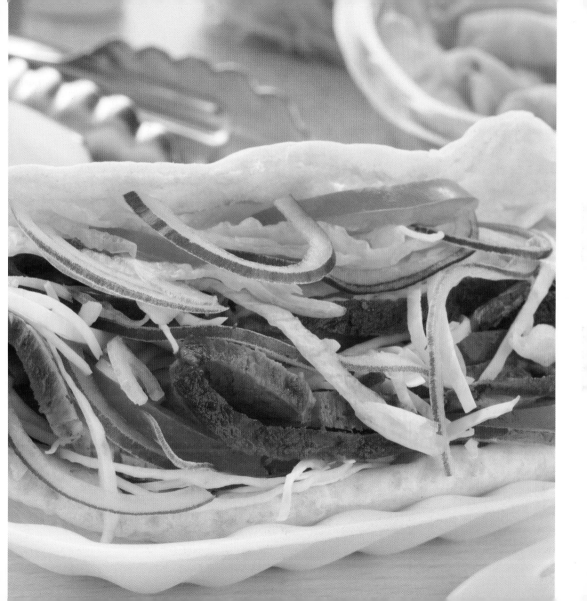

Counting Calories: Takeaway & Convenience Food

	Typical portion	Typical portion size	Calories per portion	Calories per 100 g/ml	Fat per 100 g/ml	Health rating (1–10)
Full house, regular, medium	1 slice	88 g/3⅛ oz	208	**236**	8.9	3
Ham and pineapple, 6", frozen	1	170 g/6 oz	338	**199**	4.5	3
Ham, mushroom and tomato	½	150 g/5 oz	309	**206**	4.1	3
Hawaiian, regular, medium	1 slice	88 g/3⅛ oz	196	**223**	7.3	3
Hot and spicy, regular	1 slice	88 g/3⅛ oz	204	**232**	7.6	3
Meat-topped, average	½	245 g/8⅔ oz	625	**255**	10.3	3
Mexican hot, regular	1 slice	88 g/3⅛ oz	214	**243**	9.1	3
Vegetarian, average	½	230 g/8⅛ oz	267	**216**	6.9	3

Fast Food Drinks and Ices – *see* Milk, Beverages, Desserts, pages 42, 206 and 224–26

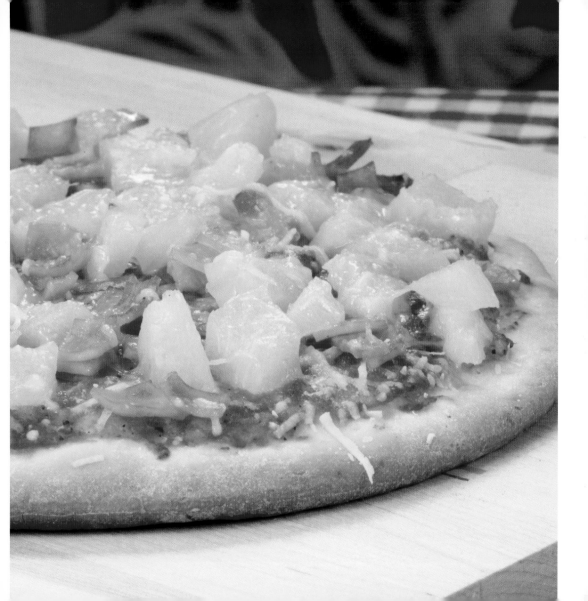

Index

Counting Calories